Medical Necessity

Medical Necessity

Health Care Access and the Politics of Decision Making

Daniel Skinner

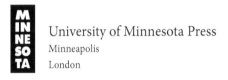

University of Minnesota Press
Minneapolis
London

Portions of chapter 5 were previously published as "The Politics of Medical Necessity in American Abortion Debates," *Politics and Gender* 8, no. 1 (2012): 1–24. DOI: 10.1017/S17439 23X12000050

Published by the University of Minnesota Press
111 Third Avenue South, Suite 290
Minneapolis, MN 55401-2520
http://www.upress.umn.edu

Printed in the United States of America on acid-free paper

The University of Minnesota is an equal-opportunity educator and employer.

Library of Congress Cataloging-in-Publication Data
Names: Skinner, Daniel, author.
Title: Medical necessity : health care access and the politics of decision making / Daniel Skinner.
Description: Minneapolis : University of Minnesota Press, [2019] | Includes bibliographical references and index. |
Identifiers: LCCN 2019007796 (print) | ISBN 978-1-5179-0376-3 (hc) | ISBN 978-1-5179-0377-0 (pb)
Subjects: | MESH: Clinical Decision-Making | Politics | Needs Assessment | Gatekeeping | Insurance, Health, Reimbursement | Unnecessary Procedures | United States
Classification: LCC RA418 (print) | NLM WB 141 | DDC 362.1—dc23
LC record available at https://lccn.loc.gov/2019007796

Contents

Abbreviations

ABN	Advance Beneficiary Notice
ACA	Affordable Care Act
ADHD	Attention Deficit Hyperactivity Disorder
AMA	American Medical Association
APA	American Psychiatric Association
CMS	United States Centers for Medicare and Medicaid Services
CPT	Current Procedural Terminology
CSA	Controlled Substances Act
D&X	Dilation and Extraction
DSM	Diagnostic and Statistical Manual of Mental Disorders
E&M	Evaluation and Management
EFM	Electronic Fetal Monitoring
ERISA	Employment and Retirement Income Security Act of 1974
FDA	United States Food and Drug Administration
HCA	Hospital Corporation of America
HCPCS	Healthcare Common Procedure Coding System
HHS	United States Department of Health and Human Services
HIPAA	Health Insurance Portability and Accountability Act
HMO	Health Maintenance Organization
ICD	International Classification of Diseases, Injuries, and Causes of Death
IMRT	Intensity-Modulated Radiation Therapy
IPAB	Independent Payment Advisory Board
MCO	Managed Care Organization
MHPAEA	Mental Health Parity and Addiction Equity Act of 2008
OCBC	Oakland Cannabis Buyers' Cooperative
ODD	Oppositional Defiant Disorder
OMT	Osteopathic Manipulative Treatment
URAC	Utilization Review Accreditation Commission
VBAC	Vaginal Birth After C-Section
WHO	World Health Organization

Introduction

A Contentious Term of Medical Decision Making

For better or worse, Americans have become accustomed to their health care services being regulated by insurance companies. As such, the language of medical necessity, which serves as the central concept within these regulatory systems, is extremely familiar.[1] This familiarity owes to the ubiquitous role medical necessity plays in virtually every aspect of medical decision making within American health care. It is a key term of American health care's most basic policy documents. It is the key concept in medical institutions' financing and reimbursement schemes. Interest groups and lobbies attempt to shape it. Advocates of marginalized groups evoke it. Physicians declare it as a routine matter of their clinical assessment, from vaccination to bypass surgery to cancer therapies. Patients assert it. Yet, at the same time, it is medical necessity's ubiquity that makes it such a curious concept. Indeed, at the center of the politics of medical necessity stands a paradox—medical necessity is a well-known and often-evoked rhetoric, but we are rarely clear about its meaning.

This is not to say that we do not talk about medical necessity. To the contrary, we do so all the time. Physicians, practice managers and employees, and patients contend with insurers about the terms of medical necessity on an almost daily basis. Most Americans first confront medical necessity when insurers reject health care services ordered by doctors—whether through a preauthorization process or, more dramatically, after the procedure has already been completed. In 2018, for example, the health insurer Anthem announced its intention to bill patients if a "utilization review" determined that care they received in emergency departments was not, in fact, an emergency—even if emergency physicians believed tests or other interventions were necessary.[2] Setting aside the question of how medical necessity is determined, these kinds of policies provoke understandable frustration and concern.

Such policies undermine efforts to establish a system that can make medical necessity decision making both predictable and credible. The result is palpable distrust about the intentions and interests of those who decide medical necessity's meaning. Stakeholders may doubt, for example, that a decision was grounded in clinical evidence. The common assumption that financial concerns supersede medical judgment raises troubling possibilities for our entire understanding of the basis of American medicine itself. Americans' trust in their medical institutions remains stuck at a dismal 40 percent.[3] Perhaps of even greater concern is the steady erosion of American trust in their personal physicians.[4]

A much-discussed 2018 case played to many Americans' worst fears that medical necessity rejections may lack clinical or ethical grounding. In a way that was perfectly positioned to stoke the public's already existing preconceptions of the insurance industry, a former medical director for Aetna acknowledged under oath that he did not look closely—or, in some cases, at all—at patient's medical records when issuing denials. Aetna claimed that the former employee's comments were "taken out of context to create media and courtroom leverage, and is a gross misrepresentation of how the process actually works."[5] Aetna offered a defense of their process and the medical director clarified his comments, describing a quite detailed decision-making process, the integrity of which hung on the meaning of the words "medical record" and whether he had read the actual medical record or just a summary of key points. Other insurers were quick to claim that Aetna's practices are an anomaly and certainly not how their company operated. Despite Aetna's defense, the rhetorical effect was already in place. Media accounts had stoked public suspicion as state insurance regulators and attorneys general prepared to investigate and, if necessary, sue the company.

Beyond these often difficult and seemingly everyday patient contexts, where wellness and prevention, health and sickness, and even life and death appear to hang in the balance of a medical necessity judgment, we encounter high-profile and explicitly political cases. These clashes are driven by standard narratives such as the inherent indignity of clinical decisions made for purposes of profit, questions about patients' rights, and physician autonomy. These disagreements are deeply political—as shown by the questions we may logically find ourselves asking, questions that commonly appear in the news media: Is abortion ever medically necessary? What about gender reassignment surgery? Is marijuana for nausea or pain relief an acceptable alternative to opioids? Treatment for depression? Under what conditions could these be described as necessary? Where do we draw the line in less-clear situations? Is it possible that medical necessity is not as clear as its rhetorical façade makes it seem?

The politics of medical necessity is integral to the negotiation and establishment of priorities in American medical care. It regulates access to goods and services for individual patients, as well as the legitimacy of the processes through which this regulatory function takes place. Since health care in the United States is big money, medical necessity determinations are never far from questions of cost. Denials of medical care are, of course, never popular, but they are less so when a palpable sense of injustice underpins the decision-making process.

As we might expect, professional interests tend to resist medical necessity oversight. In 2015, the Centers for Medicare and Medicaid Services (CMS) announced that it would require doctors to attempt nonsurgical interventions before undertaking hip and knee replacement surgery. The American Orthopedic Association issued statements with politically laden language that gestured toward a heyday when medical decisions were made "between the patient and his or her doctor," but were now in the hands of government "regulators."[6] That such a heyday may be a fiction is beside the point. The problem is real, especially within the context of the utilization of scarce resources. From CMS's perspective, surgery must be "reserved for patients whose symptoms have not responded to other treatments."[7] Therefore, Medicare will not pay for joint replacements unless patients and their physicians have made documented attempts to avoid surgery. This reminds us that necessity's meaning is sometimes attenuated and adjusted not only by a sense of urgency, but by the presence of other options that may be more or less expensive, or options that are deemed more appropriate by a party, such as an insurer, with the power to make such a determination. In these cases, a patient's or physician's judgment that surgery is necessary is tempered by considerations imposed from beyond the physician–patient dyad.

The actors within medical necessity debates include patients and physicians, as I have noted, but also the pharmaceutical, hospital, and insurance industries, physicians' groups, the American Association of Retired Persons (AARP), marijuana supporters and opponents, mental health and disability rights advocates, various governmental and nongovernmental actors, and pressure groups on both the federal and state levels. The distinctions that these groups shape—health and sickness, needs and wants, ability and disability, and even life and death—are of direct consequence to both the controversial and the quotidian issues in medicine. To see medical necessity clearly, we must see such groups as formidable forces that shape the broader politics of medical necessity. These groups raise questions about whether "necessity" signifies an existential floor, such as survival, or whether it champions a more robust vision of medicine's capacity to promote human flourishing, quality of life, happiness, longevity, and other deeply political values. For example, should medical need include such increasingly popular, if trendy, contemporary notions as wellness and preventive care? Or should medical need be restricted to more rare, expensive, and even "catastrophic" needs, as David Goldhill, the author of a widely read health policy book, suggests?[8] Should reproductive health care be cast as a question of medical necessity, or as part of a more explicitly political question that draws on terms such as freedom, autonomy, or discrimination? As I illustrate through this book, the prevalence of medical necessity as a rhetorical frame arises out of American political culture itself, a great portion of which associates choice with freedom and reduces social support or government aid only to that which is deemed necessary. Some political actors argue that expansive conceptions of medical necessity facilitate overreach for purposes that they perceive as violating social norms. Such perceived overreach has led conservative forces to attempt to restrict medical necessity on cultural, religious, or traditional grounds, especially when it comes to medical interventions perceived as reworking supposedly traditional gender norms. Similarly, liberal groups may advocate for a more expansive conception of medical necessity insofar as such a conception may facilitate individual liberty or serve as a counterweight to repressive forms of social power.

Even more broadly, medical necessity debates often raise questions about the very purpose of medicine and the nature of medical subjects. This book's central contention is that an examination of medical necessity unearths political dynamics that both constrain and enable health care policymaking on a larger scale—with daily medical necessity debates collectively amounting to a persistent uncertainty about the basic mechanisms and aims of medical decision making. As such, there is a potentially lucrative payoff—metaphorically and literally—in attaining a better understanding of medical necessity's social and rhetorical dynamics. To gain such an understanding, we must consider a wide range of theoretical questions. The answers to these questions are especially critical in the United States, where insurers and medical providers use medical necessity to regulate health services while at the same time positioning themselves to shape its meaning.

Of course, the United States is not unique among the world's nations in using medical necessity as a regulatory policy tool. Thus, it is not only medical necessity's presence in policy debates that is worth noting, but *how* it appears in *specific* policy debates that is politically relevant and illuminating. Accordingly, instead of calling for a rejection of the concept of medical necessity, as some have proposed, this book pays attention to how medical necessity is deployed rhetorically, as well as the way this rhetoric is instrumentalized and threaded through disagreements within a broader politics of medicine. In doing so we can both illuminate the political and medical cultures that shape American health care debates and better understand medical necessity itself. In the chapters that follow, I demonstrate how a close reading of several case studies reveals the politics of medical necessity at work in American health policy.

Medical Necessity's Role in American Health Care

The multipayer nature of American health care magnifies the challenges of using the concept of medical necessity to regulate health care services. Specifically, the system within which most Americans encounter medical necessity determinations includes private companies with insurance plans geared toward employers and individuals; Medicare for seniors; access to Veterans Affairs services for veterans and TRICARE for active duty military; more than fifty different state and U.S. territory Medicaid plans for the poor, near poor, and disabled; a public health care program for near poor children (Children's Health Insurance Program, or CHIP); and, most recently, in the influx of Americans who gained access to private individual plans shaped by the Affordable Care Act (ACA). Despite this complex web of access points, a critical rethinking of medical necessity rarely arises within the context of health policy discussions. In health systems and health services research, the concept is usually an uninterrogated and little-noticed substratum.

Though the ACA is an important part of contemporary American health care discussions, Trump administration efforts to repeal the ACA have not drastically altered the politics of medical necessity. This is because medical necessity is as central to private insurance determinations as it is to government-financed health care. The fact that the ACA did so little to critically rethink medical necessity is both part of its authors' political savvy (for by stoking these flames such discussions would likely have forestalled broader reform efforts aimed at expanding access) as well as a symptom of how little the ACA did to rework fundamental questions about health care in the United States. The ACA's benefits to American patients came primarily through an expansion of the basic systems already in place, and did not radically overhaul the nation's overarching approach to health care.

Even the adoption of single-payer universal health care in the United States, which would further expand access to health care services, would not necessarily settle the question of medical necessity. This is not to say, of course, that universal health care couldn't, in principle, engage the question of medical necessity, but rather that the politics of addressing the meaning of necessity would likely be a different politics than that which accompanies expanded access. A critical engagement with medical necessity requires rethinking medicine's conceptual foundations—such as what constitutes disease, or what is and is not considered necessary to attain wellness—rather than merely expanding existing foundations, which are often a source of problems instead of solutions. If anything, expanded access should provide a reason for thinking more seriously about the meaning of medical necessity, which, as I show throughout this book, requires critically rethinking larger value sets. The budgetary consequences of expansion alone, where unclear terms can be costly, would likely force the issue. The fact that this has not been the case tells us something important about medical necessity as it is understood within the context of American health care politics, namely that Americans and their political representatives clearly do not wish to take on issues at the core of the politics of medical necessity.

Paradoxically, the stakes of the politics of medical necessity are not particularly high for one important group within American health care: the uninsured. Of course, we should be concerned with what the uninsured need—such a concern, after all, driven by moral and civic concern, is central to health care reform. The arrival of a single-payer system would likely have tremendous benefits for uninsured Americans, yet such benefits would not be a result of any substantial systemic changes concerning medical necessity. This disjunction between the uninsured and medical necessity underscores the fact that the very existence of a medical necessity rejection presumes that a patient has health coverage in the first place.[9] The medical needs of this population are simply ignored within these debates.

One notable exception is emergency care, which remains generally reliable in the United States, at least for the documented, in large part because the Emergency Medical Treatment and Labor Act requires that U.S. emergency departments care for patients to a point of stabilization. Some questions do of course exist at the margins of American health care politics regarding the nature of medical necessity in emergencies. David Cone and colleagues, for example, have sought to bring expert consensus to bear on establishing medical necessity criteria for emergency medical services.[10] There is, as well, a large and growing literature that addresses strategies for reducing medically unnecessary emergency department use.[11] Other studies explore the role that new models, such as shared decision making, can play in determining with greater accuracy and appropriateness whether a patient should be admitted to emergency departments.[12] In general, however, the state of medical services for uninsured populations, beyond the declaration of an emergency, exceeds the scope of this book. Instead, I focus primarily on questions posed by determinations made for individuals with health coverage. The question of what to do with someone who asserts medical necessity but has no access to health care services is a broader question of human rights. Other scholars have taken up this question within this context, including the role that medical claims may play when political appeals—such as asylum and persecution claims—do not work.[13]

What kind of political dynamics are at work within the politics of medical necessity as they play out in a system in which third parties—especially insurers and governments—must make distinctions between the necessary and unnecessary? Taxpayer funded national health care programs, as I have noted, do not circumvent the politics of medical necessity simply by removing profit motives from medical decision making; rather, they shift the debate to a different plane. Observers of health care are aware of a similar dynamic in some of our most pressing challenges, where a refined—and not merely expanded—conception of medical necessity is critical to making health insurance plans more evidence-based. The development of such criteria is an important step toward ensuring that, for example, end of life care is not merely an opportunity for profiteering on the part of unscrupulous providers who stand to benefit from unnecessary surgeries and other medical interventions. The news is filled with similar such reports.[14]

There are many ways in which medical necessity can be misrepresented, misinterpreted, and turned into a profit center instead of a clinical foundation. Yet, the United States has not positioned itself well to engage or challenge such instances. Indeed, one of the great puzzles of American health care politics is how major policy developments have not brought us closer to settling the question of medical necessity's meaning. Just as noteworthy is that none of the actors—especially legislative actors— involved in these developments have made a serious attempt to try. This failure to engage medical necessity in a sustained and serious manner has left the American health care system vulnerable as clinically insecure grounds leave patients open to confusion and even predation.

Could this reluctance to engage the question be the result of an assumption that these determinations remain a clinician's prerogative? Or is it an awareness of the political dangers of engaging the powerful interest groups that are likely to resist such efforts? This reluctance to engage the question likely speaks to something fundamental about medical necessity itself: a combination of the political stakes it represents and its conceptual amorphousness. The very nature of this concept makes agreement difficult and even unattractive for some key stakeholders.

From an engagement with medical coding, which captures a general challenge posed by medical necessity, to the specific cases of marijuana, mental health, and reproduction, we must reread medical necessity debates in an explicitly political manner. This requires that we approach those debates with an eye toward understanding commonly deployed strategies within qualitatively different medical necessity debates. It requires spanning a wide range of questions, from the problems inherent in depoliticized definitional debates and legal challenges to openly political approaches centered on the needs of marginalized populations, populations with specific health care needs, and the intersection of a politics animated by different moral and medical perspectives. It requires investigating medical necessity's philosophical roots, which illuminate the concept's significance as a policy tool, as well as its pragmatic and rhetorical deployment in policy debates.

Medical Necessity, Rhetoric, and Power

This book argues that medical necessity decision making takes place within fields of power that both limit and expand medical necessity's scope. An analysis of discursive structures is one important way that we can begin to observe, understand, and critique these power relations. When one takes note of the specific axes of power in disagreements over medical necessity's terms, one reveals the qualitative differences that distinguish various medical questions from one another. In some cases, medical necessity will appear as a purely clinical question, with differing views on clinical appropriateness driving the debate. At other times the question arises as a primarily legal one. In many of these cases, identity structures such as gender play a key role, showing the extent to which men, women, and gender-nonconforming individuals are located within medical regimes that carry with them their own conceptions of necessity. Some medical necessity debates reveal disagreement about the word *medical* itself, which is given meaning not only by intrinsic valuation, but also by external forces, such as neoliberal economics and conservative conceptions of the body. These debates underscore the extent to which the medical is given meaning by what some theorists call constitutive others, such as the cosmetic, the recreational, the experimental, and other rhetorical markers of nonnecessity.

The discursive forces and rhetorical practices within the politics of medical necessity raise fundamental questions of fairness, tend to be organized hierarchically, and are especially noticeable along lines of gender, sexuality, race, ability, and class. For example, questions concerning the medical necessity of woman's reproductive choices tend to be treated more skeptically by policy makers and are subject to more intense forms of elite power in comparison to the areas of mental health or marijuana. The rhetoric of choice stands in clear opposition to the rhetoric of medical necessity, as does the rhetoric of freedom—all of which play an important role in the debates this book explores.

Race, as we would expect, plays an important role in shaping the degree of trust that people have in medical institutions that make medical necessity determinations. It is well known, for example, that African Americans distrust medical institutions at higher rates than whites, a deficit that is directed at physicians as well as the larger medical systems in which physicians are located.[15] Predictably, disagreements about medical necessity tend to have consequences for justice and fairness and are almost always encumbered by the specter of discrimination. A political analysis of medical necessity requires an investigation of how these arguments are constructed and where lines are drawn, and a better understanding of why some medical choices gain the legitimacy medical necessity bestows, while others do not.

The specific mechanisms through which medical necessity debates are constituted is of primary importance. These mechanisms include metaphors, argument structures, warrants from or appeals to logic and reason, metaphysical assertions, and assumptions. It is on the level of rhetoric that medical necessity's politics are most vividly observable, not only in formal documents, but in expressions and defenses of physicians' and patients' views, theoretical works on necessity, and the documents that comprise legal challenges to medical necessity denials.

Throughout this book I draw upon two distinct scholarly lenses: Foucauldian conceptions of power and rhetorical analysis. Both may be presumed to be in the background of my analysis, even when I do not specifically evoke them. Despite their quite different ways of engaging the dimensions of power and knowledge that are critical to medical necessity, each opens important spaces for undertaking a theoretical investigation of the concept.

Power

Power stabilizes itself by policing attempts to undermine the knowledge claims that sustain it. Michel Foucault famously captures this dynamic through a theoretical innovation he calls power/knowledge. It is in defense of systems of power/knowledge that challenges to existing truths—such as nonconventional and nonelite viewpoints, or lay conceptions of medical necessity—are disciplined and resisted. Accordingly, in contemporary health care certain assumptions may be deemed true because they accord with neoliberal orthodoxies circulating in social and political life, such as presumptions about resource scarcity, the sustainability of systems, or the deservedness of patients who may be underemployed or unemployed. Similarly, patient behaviors are often refracted through conventional wisdoms, such as those concerning "noncompliance" or frivolous lawsuits that are assumed to be unavoidable by the physician. This neoliberal discourse leaves in its wake a pathology of unreasonable, lazy, or "litigious" patients.[16] Because this conventional wisdom, with accompanying rhetoric, has ossified within our broader politics, it is often difficult to critically rethink it.[17] As a medical educator, I have observed how these discourses are deeply lodged in the very socialization of medical students as well. To some degree, these assumptions unhelpfully reinforce the identity of the besieged physician who is losing control over medical judgment—precisely as Foucault would expect.

Cast within a Foucauldian framework, medical necessity is not a privileged domain of one medical actor repressing or shaping another (as when a physician is thought to have power over a patient), but the negotiations and contestations of multiple forces within a network, in which actors are best understood as what Foucault calls "vehicles" or transmitters of power. The forces that shape medical necessity are themselves subject to this diffuse distribution of power. The question is not only who gets to decide when something is medically necessary, but how myriad forces simultaneously shape medical necessity's discursive boundaries and how they themselves are then shaped by those same boundaries.

Rhetoric and Persuasion

Where the Foucauldian view of the relationship between discursive power and rhetoric departs is in the rhetorical tradition's general view, at least since Aristotle, that rhetoric is an art primarily concerned with identifying and understanding the tools for persuasion in different contexts and for different aims.[18] In the Aristotelian view, one would deploy quite different rhetorical tools as a physician trying to persuade a patient or a patient trying to persuade an insurance company than a lawyer would in trying to persuade a jury, or a teacher would in trying to persuade a student.

Rhetoric scholars have, at least since Plato, tended to conceptualize persuasion as incompatible with force, which is a formidable part of medical power.[19] The traditional view of rhetoric requires that one be open to persuasion regardless of the contexts of power within which one is situated, as when new evidence arises about the nonnecessity of certain tests, or where necessity can be established persuasively in previously contested spaces. As such, an emphasis on persuasion champions an openness that is essential to civic life but that often sits uncomfortably alongside claims to objectivity created through primarily biomedical models. In contrast, as Foucault notes, "orders of discourse" become entrenched in systems of power, are disciplined and entrenched through the repetition of discourse, and are taught as "true." They are challenged not through counterdiscourses that are regarded ultimately as persuasive, which would suggest that social knowledge is purely rational, but because they are overthrown through protracted struggles. This "insurrection of subjugated knowledges"[20] changes the terms of existing regimes of power/knowledge through contestation and agitation, not persuasion.

Foucault wisely downplays persuasion's capacity to alter power. This is especially the case to the extent that what is or is not persuasive is a function of power/knowledge. My turn to rhetoric, however, is motivated by two supplemental positions. First, rhetorical analysis provides a means of understanding power/knowledge to the extent that analyzing the internal coherency (or lack thereof) of knowledge claims can expose the legitimacy of those claims. In a way, this approach draws upon a method of questioning as much as it does rhetorical analysis, particularly since it uses the exposure of internal contradiction to evaluate and potentially destabilize truth claims. Second, exposing cracks in the rhetorical structure of truth provides an opening for contesting them. Rhetoric's persuasive capacities may be insufficient for contesting power, but the tools of rhetorical analysis are helpful for understanding how discursive regimes are constructed, as well as for mounting challenges. It is the spirit of this approach that I draw on in my readings of medical coding, marijuana, mental health, and reproduction.

As we read, we must also calibrate our expectations. After all, it would be unreasonable to expect that what Foucault calls an "insurrection" would lead to the complete and sudden overthrow of an order of discourse, such as an existing approach toward medical necessity or the reversal of conventional medical wisdom. Instead, we should expect change to occur through the slow boring of holes and exploiting of cracks in knowledge, where the previously unnecessary can be altered and that which previously seemed necessary to cure disease or improve health can be exposed as unjustified or even dangerous. Is there not in such discourses a persuasive component, as when a legitimizing foundation of power/knowledge begins to fray because it is no longer believable or sustainable?

The combination of rhetoric and Foucauldian power allows us to notice not only what kinds of claims are made about medical necessity, but also how they are constructed. Indeed, a primary goal of such an approach is precisely to be *able* to see medical necessity as constructed. My turn toward rhetorical analysis is intended to provide readers with a means of reading, in a critical manner, the truth that underpins medical necessity claims. In one sense, this approach is not a departure from Foucault. Foucauldian methodologies and rhetoric are, in fact, symbiotic if one closely aligns rhetoric with Foucault's evocation of "discourse" as a means by which knowledge is constructed and maintained within power/knowledge.[21] If one follows Foucault in taking seriously Nietzsche's view of truth as "a mobile army of metaphors, metonyms, anthropomorphisms, in short, a sum of human relations which were poetically and rhetorically heightened," then one is situated to see truths about medicine, patients, clinicians, and beyond as rhetorically packaged subjects of power.[22] Things came full circle when Foucault, in his later years, begins to speak of "games of truth" instead of regimes. This move gestures toward the metaphors that one more commonly finds in rhetorical and critical language theory, from Wittgensteinian "language games" to Derridean "play,"[23] though we should not let these metaphors cast doubt on the seriousness of the question. Health professionals of various stripes routinely characterize the need to prove medical necessity for reimbursement as a game that impedes their ability to care for patients.

Politics

This book attempts to balance controversial questions of medical necessity with those that tend to go unnoticed. While I discuss medical marijuana, for example, I also discuss mental and behavioral health, where questions about medical necessity tend to be subtler. Since medical necessity debates often center on controversial questions concerning sexuality and gender, I attend to these threads throughout, with a recognition that these distinct concepts are intricately bound up in power relations that shape virtually all medical necessity decision making. Abortion, in particular, has been a contentious area in which actors have evoked medical necessity, often as a way to neutralize arguments about the beginning of life and the politics of choice.[24] But just as important are the subtler, less conspicuous areas in which debates over the meaning of medical necessity arise. To an extent, the politics of medical necessity is a politics of nuanced dynamics and tactical rhetorical positioning—something that medical necessity scholars rarely seem to notice, not to mention debate.

A dynamic rethinking of medical necessity requires approaching it as a form of partial knowledge inscribed in living and fluid documents.[25] Since these definitional questions play out in various political theaters, references to real or actual medical necessity are not only insufficient, but likely to further entrench uninterrogated medical necessity definitions. For example, as one news report notes, "vision correction is not deemed medically necessary. . . . A detached retina is a different matter." Similarly, "teeth cleaning and cavity filling are not deemed medically necessary. . . . Dental surgery is a different matter." The proof of this difference lies in the fact that "when someone had his front teeth knocked out in an accident, medical insurance paid." Complicating all of this is the question of documentation, as access to these services often depends upon "how the doc writes it up."[26] Indeed, as I show, the politics of medical necessity is largely a politics of writing.

What may appear to be a simple question of categorizing and codifying care is actually a complex question of valuation, body politics, identity politics, and biomedical ethics. These questions are not limited to obvious areas of disagreement, such as those raised about the medical necessity of abortion, sleeping pills, or the removal of excess skin after weight loss.[27] Even a surgeon's decision to leave a metal wire inside a patient under general anesthesia—where medical necessity arises at the margins of malpractice—can sometimes travel under the sign of medical necessity.[28] Medical necessity not only serves as a gatekeeper to care, but mediates legal relations and justifies controversial decisions made by physicians when patients are not able to make their preferences known.

Medical necessity's cultural reach extends beyond questions of medical care. For example, disability law makes medical necessity a lever capable of forcing landlords to allow helping dogs so that epileptics—and others with various needs—can live in otherwise "no pet" rentals.[29] When the federal government established new passenger screening protocols after 9/11, medical necessity played a role in establishing exceptions, showing the concept's ability to penetrate the security state. In a quite different example, when polygamist leader Warren Jeffs, who was convicted of molesting children, refused to eat, courts established that Jeffs could be force fed if it was deemed medically necessary.[30] In 2013, as detainees at the American prison at Guantanamo Bay refused to eat in protest of their conditions of imprisonment and denial of due process, the same argument was made, if not out of genuine care for the detainees, then to avoid the embarrassment of protesting detainees dying under American watch in occupied Cuban territory.[31] A 2014 CIA report documented forced "rectal feeding" and other violations of international law in CIA-run prison camps, where the critics pointed to a lack of medical necessity as a reason why such acts could amount to the possible commission of torture.[32]

Within the politics of medical necessity, we find consultants advising—even coaching—physicians and their staffs on the best ways to pass unwounded through labyrinthine coding systems. We find physicians' groups advising on how to ensure that physicians are paid when their services appear to be of marginal medical necessity, but nonetheless require the legitimacy of medical necessity discourse to secure payment. Understanding the politics of medical necessity requires taking note of news stories, social media postings, and comments where many of these everyday encounters are archived and where the obscure and exceptional tend to be the norm. Reading medical necessity in this way allows us to capture the concept's exceptional and extraordinary uses as well as those that may be considered commonplace. This approach also allows us to cast medical necessity decision making as a political—instead of merely medical, technical, or scientific—debate. In line with the traditional aims of rhetoric, this recasting requires an understanding of the depth of medical necessity's cultural, political, and economic reach, as well as a rethinking of the meaning and scope of politics.

In casting medical necessity as a dynamic political concept, this book engages the question of whether medical necessity's meaning has done little more than expand as American health care has developed. Considering the typical patient's response when confronted with medical necessity rejections, and the tendency to advocate for a broader understanding, it is easy to see why this belief would be so common. Scholars offer several explanations as to why they believe it has expanded. Some critics argue that medical necessity's scope is a function of misaligned and even "perverse" incentives among health care providers and payers. In *Catastrophic Care*, for example, Goldhill argues that "the definition of health care 'need' has expanded relentlessly," a trend which he attributes in large part to financial incentives resulting from "well-intended" but misguided social policy that aimed to ensure that all patients had access to expansive health care services.[33] Goldhill's continual use of quotation marks to call need into question tells us most of what we need to know about his position. That the result of increased access to health care with powerful pressure groups advocating for expanded need would lead to an expansion of medical necessity's meaning seems obvious to Goldhill—as are the exploding costs that accompany such an expansion. After all, as Goldhill argues, again with quotation marks to denote skepticism, "all 'needed' care must be paid for."[34] In Goldhill's telling, this inflated sense of need is an effect of a conflation and misunderstanding of the differences between health—which encompasses first order variables such as exercise and diet—and health care. I return to this theme in subsequent chapters since it brings a critical view of the meaning of the "medical" into focus. Particularly important to note, however, is that Goldhill rightly notes that how we define medical necessity has direct consequences on whether the American health care system is sustainable. The same is true regarding what is ultimately considered to be a medical issue and what is not, what we consider to be within the scope of medicine's reach and what is beyond it, and what we wish to ascribe to deeper, more expansive social dynamics and what we wish to identify with or locate in individual persons and patients.

Each of the following chapters reveals something important about the politics of health and medicine in the United States. This is because, in the United States, broad discussions about health promotion tend to raise concerns, especially but not exclusively from conservatives, about liberty as it is affected by social policy. Serious considerations about the meaning of necessity, or what one needs, militate against the rhetoric of choice, or what one wants or one's ability to determine what one needs for oneself. Institutions and traditions, both of which are imbued with power, constrain necessity as well as choice. While few public health advocates would like to see medical necessity determined in the abstract, as part of a large-scale, algorithm-driven administrative project, a broad and ongoing discussion about the modes of decision making that underpin American health care utilization is illuminating.

Structure of the Argument

While the cases I engage in chapters 2 through 5 are where we see medical necessity in action, and where I engage its politics most substantively, some degree of theoretical and historical background is necessary before undertaking these analyses. A key part of the politics of necessity is precisely that the concept is undertheorized and rarely even noticed, despite its ubiquity in American health care policy. Accordingly, chapter 1 explores the theoretical foundations of necessity, with attention to key developments that led to the rise of medical necessity as a gatekeeper concept in American health care. After discussing problems associated with approaching medical necessity as a purely definitional matter, I present this history by breaking down the perspectives of various actors participating in medical necessity decision making: patients, physicians, payers, and appeals processes. Chapter 1 also offers readers a brief history of medical necessity told through the different perspectives brought to bear by physicians, patients, payers, and within appeals processes, each of which reminds us that different actors have different interests.

To understand the formative role that medical necessity plays in shaping medical knowledge and discourse within American health care, chapter 2 explores the industry of schools, publications, and computer software that has arisen to meet the challenges medical necessity poses to coding for reimbursement, making coding a burgeoning trade that is often cast as an exciting and profitable employment opportunity within the health care sector. By engaging medical coding, this chapter shows that largely unresolvable paradoxes within the politics of medical necessity reside at the foundations of American health care's approach to financing. This makes medical necessity not only an important term of qualitative distinction, but one of financial and fiscal import as well. Yet, this turn to medical necessity as an attempt to systematize medical financing is premised on a faulty view of language. Given the misunderstood nature of medical necessity, the result is an always frustrating, often comical, but also sometimes tragic daily attempt to capture medical necessity within existing and evolving coding schemas. It is, as medical coding trainers will often admit, a game.

Chapters 2 through 5 examine the centrality of the politics of medical necessity within three specific controversies over medical coverage and treatment. These chapters take readers through a series of politically and medically contentious issues, each of which offers a distinct analytic lens on medical necessity. Each of these lenses, moreover, evokes a different rhetorical dimension within medical necessity's broader politics and explores a qualitatively different question for the politics of medical necessity itself.

Medical marijuana debates, the focus of chapter 3, challenge not only the meaning of medical necessity, but the political value of so-called medical necessity defenses. Such defenses show the extent to which medical necessity can operate as a legal or quasi-legal discourse, and illustrate medical necessity's ability to shield marijuana users from the complexities of, and tensions within, federal and state marijuana laws. The chapter's key takeaway is the extent to which the rhetoric of medical necessity can be viewed as a legal question, its rhetorical reach threading through court cases and statutes. In American medical marijuana debates, legal categories tarry with political categories, and the medical tarries with a persistent skepticism that it is being evoked as cover for recreation. The case of marijuana expands our understanding of the terms of discourse that accompany medical necessity, with the necessary/unnecessary binary expanding to challenge the legitimacy of marijuana advocates' claims that the plant provides medical benefits.

Building on the discussion of marijuana, chapter 4 advances our understanding of the politics through which the boundaries of the medical are contested and reworked. Specifically, this chapter examines the intersection of medical necessity and mental health. Mental health is an important space from which to study medical necessity because it tends to evoke disagreement about the boundaries between "normal" life struggles and problems in need of clinical or other expert attention. Here I emphasize how debates over the medicalization of mental health, as well as those who challenge the viability of certain categories within mental health, impact its relationship with medical necessity decision making. This chapter complicates medical necessity's epistemic basis by evoking different standards for mental health issues than those that are generally applied to physical, bodily health issues. While marijuana debates often veer off course from debates over the meaning of the medical, mental health continues to play a key role in clarifying—by expanding as well as contracting, depending on the politics—the medicine's conceptual boundaries. Whereas negotiations of the medical/recreational distinction reside at the center of marijuana debates, mental health tends to raise questions that are both deeply social (as when mental health needs are seen as personal failures or problems stemming from "normal" life) and concerned with insurance reimbursement (as when payers attempt to limit the scope of the medical to restrict access to hard to see and protracted mental health services). Accordingly, debates about medical necessity in mental health play important roles in delineating the epistemic boundaries of medicine more generally.

Broadening our understanding of the boundaries of the medical, chapter 5 examines the intersection of gendered social power and medical necessity. Specifically, it examines the confluence of medical necessity and reproductive politics where gender intersects with and complicates definitional debates. First, I examine research on rising American C-section rates over the past decades, which not only spotlights the intersection of the medicalization of childbirth and medical necessity but raises questions about whether medical necessity is rhetorically arranged around babies, delivering mothers, both, or—perhaps more ominously—neither. Second, to capture a quite different though related set of questions about gender and medical necessity, I review the protracted history of medical necessity discourse in American abortion debates. Here medical necessity is cast as an existential floor, a way out of the rancorous theater of American abortion politics in which debates about specific procedures or the definition of life are exchanged for an argument about the life or health of the pregnant woman. I argue that deflecting the political debate by turning to the medical has far-reaching consequences for the politics of abortion. In thinking about C-section and abortion together, I show medical necessity's rhetorical double-edge in reproductive politics, where medical discourse is evoked as both a means of defending women's rights in some cases (the right to have an abortion) but also as a means of limiting their options in childbirth (in the case of C-section).

Taken together, these chapters show why definitional debates are inherently political, but also the qualitatively different ways in which each conceptual question arises. From the broader theoretical contours of medical necessity to its specific role in contentious political theaters, I show both why medical necessity is an important question for social scientists to consider and how a close analysis of it can illuminate important dynamics within some of the most contentious medical, and political, questions of our time.

The conclusion explores strategies for rethinking the rhetoric of medical necessity. Because of the epistemological questions a critique of medical necessity raises, I question the wisdom of operationalizing medical necessity when thinking critically about some of our most vexing health care challenges. I do this by exploring three strategies that could play a role in seeing our way through the contentious politics of medical necessity: contracts, rights, and technology. Though each strategy is rhetorically attractive in its own way, I describe the significant limitations that preclude each from resolving the problems that this book identifies. Ultimately, I explain, depoliticizing rhetorical strategies such as those associated with contracts, rights, or technological solutions is unlikely to resolve the debates at the center of the politics of medical necessity. Worse yet, it might serve to muddy rather than clarify our understanding.

With these false hopes in mind, and conceding that medical necessity will remain central to American health care politics at least for the near future, the book concludes with a defense of an overtly political approach to medical necessity. This approach acknowledges that medical necessity is the product of strategic positioning and agitation by key stakeholders. While these stakeholders may attempt to secure their position by deploying a rhetoric of objective necessity, a critical analysis of medical necessity requires that we see beyond this. I argue not only that the politics of medical necessity is unlikely to be resolved by a new or better definition, but that such a resolution would not be desirable due to the depoliticizing effects such an attempt would have on the epistemic foundations of medical care itself. In short, in the case of medical necessity, it may be preferable to see it as a discourse, to notice the rhetorical sleights of hand and metaphysics of language at work when it is conjured within the broader context of American health care politics. What we lose in giving up the belief that medical necessity is or can be objectively fixed, we gain in being able to engage it directly. This is particularly important for groups engaging questions of medical necessity as part of social justice projects or in the name of vulnerable populations and persons.

The problem is not the politicization of medical care, but the depoliticizing tendency to treat medical necessity decision making as a matter of facts to be found rather than sets of values to be defended. The turn to rhetoric should serve as a reminder of this view's insufficiency and each chapter addresses a piece of the broader puzzle before the summative assessment and prospective vision I offer in the conclusion. What becomes medically necessary, in the final picture, is best seen not as a mere byproduct of scientific or clinical determinations, but as an effect of advocacy, organization, and agitation. Even the relatively simple act of filing a medical necessity appeal is part of this political view, though, as I note, appeals require resources and time that many patients and physicians do not have. The key is to understand the politics of medical necessity decision making as a contest over the terms of discourse, where the result of such contests is, above all, the right to define. A different politics of medical necessity is therefore sought not by unearthing medical necessity's truth, but by a more inclusive and openly normative political process.

If we can take on this difficult question of norms and realize that medical decision making is bound up in wide-ranging social values and discourses, then we will be better positioned to think both critically and productively about medical necessity. The result is a framework for understanding medical necessity that keeps questions of power and the values inscribed in medical knowledge visible so that they may be engaged directly.

1

Medical Necessity?

A Definitional, Philosophical, and Historical Question

A critical engagement with medical necessity must grapple with the fact that rhetoric is deeply embedded in our medical forms of life, almost to a point of invisibility. If successful, a sustained critique of medical necessity will ensure that the concept never appears simple or unproblematic again. Such a critique helps us recognize the important role medical necessity plays in constituting medical subjects and in regulating an entire order of medical discourse. Such a critique will both complicate and demystify the concept. Accordingly, before turning to concrete examples we must orient ourselves to the concept itself and consider the best way to approach medical necessity as a scholarly inquiry.

Defining Medical Necessity

One might reasonably ask: if medical necessity is such a problem, why can't we just convene a committee of experts to define it and be done? While this would of course be contentious—we can already hear the objections of "Death panel!"—the limitations of such an approach run deeper than that. Specifically, medical necessity's value-laden, perspectival nature removes the possibility of locating a neutral position to which one can default. This is true even within, and perhaps even *especially* in, appeals to professional elites like physicians and biomedical researchers—whose expertise is often thought to be a sufficient final judgment. The American Medical Association, for example, tends to advocate, as one might predict, for a greater weight for physicians' voices in medical necessity determinations. They wish to empower their constituents with the right to define. Similarly, device companies and pharmaceutical representatives advocate for the expansive medical necessity of their products with office visits, presentations to clinicians (often plying them with free lunches), and advertising. There are no unproblematic voices in these debates, even as each voice may, despite self-interest, have something important to contribute to the broader debate. Indeed, given the inherent politics of definition, working constructively with self-interested advocates may be the only viable option.

This is in large part because to settle on a definition is to take a position on the matter of value. As rhetoric scholars have long argued, when one privileges certain voices, one privileges a perspective. This effect is present when that privileged perspective is grounded in a review of clinical evidence or when assumptions are based on perceptions stemming from professional training or institutional position, like the trust that so many Americans place in their physicians. Though we may wish to regard such a perspective as "right," the key point is to recognize that such legitimacy is a function of the role that politics plays in medical necessity decision making. The politics of medical necessity is, among other things, a function of persuasive effects.

Questions of medical necessity concern varying conceptions of the meaning of a quality life, subjective calculations of value in using resources that are perceived to be scarce, the intersections of religion, culture, and medical intervention—and a wide range of other economic and social questions. The key considerations tend to be: what limits do individuals and institutions put on the meaning of necessity, and what are necessity's ends? In other words: necessary for what?

The ability of a neutral or objective perspective to arise in medical necessity decision making is a rhetorical sleight of hand. The arrival of such a perspective confuses our ability to understand what is actually taking place.[1] Some scholars have even conceptualized a "rhetoric of neutrality" in creating the appearance of value-neutrality in value-laden systems.[2] To be sure, there are reasons why certain forms of knowledge come to be naturalized as real, normal, or true. Such forms of knowledge, which Foucault called "epistemes," take hold because they accord with dominant systems of power/knowledge and are therefore circulated, repeated, recited, and evoked until they appear fixed and even natural. But this naturalization, it is important to note, is also a rhetorical effect, even when it appears that the knowledge at hand is well founded. The first step to understanding medical necessity therefore requires jettisoning the pretense of timeless description, the metaphysics of which take us afield from, instead of closer to, understanding medical necessity within the context of medical power.

The first methodological point to be made about medical necessity is that it is contextual precisely where universal definitions are made possible through a process of decontextualization. Neutrality and objectivity only become possible in the absence of context.

A thornier issue concerns the political nature of definition itself. As Raymond Williams has noted, while dictionaries may fix meanings, contested and essentially contestable concepts that "involve ideas and values" make definition "not only impossible but an irrelevant procedure."[3] Worse than being irrelevant, such an approach may divert us from the phenomena at hand, depositing us in a circular language game instead of positioning us to think clearly about the values that we wish to govern the utilization of health care services. A political reading of medical necessity requires not simply joining the chorus of normative argument as to what should and what should not be considered medically necessary or seeking to uncover it from existing criteria, but approaching definition itself as a political question, with attention to the power to define.

Such a turn underscores the extent to which legitimacy is a persuasive effect, in this case largely owing to the credibility of those empowered to define. Turning to certain individuals or institutions in such a way is akin to entrusting them with accessing a certain truth, such as the properly or purely medical. Of course, what we might call the "properly" or "purely" medical is always itself a fiction, a proxy for other discourses. For example, medical discourses are often also educational discourses, educational discourses are often penal discourses, penal discourses are moral, and so on.[4]

Sara Singer and Linda Bergthold, two prominent scholars of medical necessity, note that "the decision-making *process* itself is in need of improvement."[5] This reminds us that since medical necessity cannot be defined in the abstract, one of the most important dimensions of the politics of medical necessity regards process and procedures, as well as the values—transparency, especially—that accompany them. This procedural turn moves our inquiry to the domain of legal challenges to medical necessity decision-making appeals, which comprise moral as well as legal appeals. We must evaluate this process while exploring the dispositions of and roles played by key actors. To assume this perspective is to acknowledge that medical necessity's history is composed of "conflict over meanings and attempts by various groups to gain public support for their particular view and for the 'facts' that they claim about it."[6]

The libertarian scholar E. Haavi Morreim describes medical necessity as "notoriously difficult, if not impossible, to define." Somewhat less descriptively, he adds that it is composed of "clinical artificiality," which undercuts attempts to "say that one option is 'necessary' . . . while the other is 'unnecessary,'" a distinction that Morreim seeks to establish credibly, though it is not clear how this is to be accomplished. His solution is to deflect the question. Since no necessary–unnecessary distinction is obviously "correct," Morreim raises a question about ends, asserting that medical necessity can only be "defined relative to a goal." He concludes, "To presume that a medical intervention is objectively either necessary or unnecessary belies the legitimacy of such variation in human goals and values."[7] From this perspective, all fixed points that supposedly ground medical necessity determinations are revealed to be functions of larger value-sets.

Other prominent libertarians acknowledge the relationship between ethos and value. Building on Morreim's critique of necessity, for example, Michael Cannon, the libertarian Cato Institute's director of health policy studies, emphasizes the question of authority. He notes, for example, that "the question becomes: who will do a better job of deciding whether and when hip replacements or antibiotics or Viagra are 'medically necessary?' Regulators? Or patients choosing health plans (in part) based on how those plans define medical necessity?"[8] In an attempt to circumvent the problem of authority by exchanging authority in defining medical necessity for patient choice in selecting plans, Cannon suggests that if the terms of medical necessity decision making were spelled out in greater detail within insurance contracts patients would be able to choose a better plan. This view assumes, of course, that patients read and can understand such contracts, and that contracts can—presumably through clearly written terms and careful attention to the deployment of concepts—establish clear criteria for medical necessity decision making. Cannon assumes that more choice will lead to more transparency in medical necessity when it is not clear that one follows from the other.

These questions suggest a need to reconsider the methods by which medical necessity is defined. We need to highlight the political contests through which medical necessity assumes a social character. "It is," after all, as Wittgenstein notes, "what human beings say that is true and false; and they agree in the language they use."[9] Wittgenstein underscores the fact that linguistic communities share an overlapping array of discursive structures. Medical necessity is a shared discourse within American medicine, but this does not mean that we share meanings as we would, for example, if stable meanings could be assured by a sovereign.[10]

One possibility scholars do not seem to entertain is that medical necessity's usefulness as a concept is a *result* of its indeterminacy. Though I return to this point in the conclusion, some preliminary comments are in order. As with all concepts at the center of policy apparatuses, it is the concept's malleability and applicability to multiple situations that make it useful. Medical necessity's context-dependence and interpretability are among the features that make it both useful and problematic as a gatekeeper concept for care. These features, of course, all give rise to the contentious politics that arises around those concepts—though we would not expect all concepts to evoke the rancor and emotion that medical necessity does. What needs to be underscored is that it should not be surprising that "attempts to achieve consensus on the meaning of medical necessity are likely to fail."[11]

Beyond the essential contestability of concepts, specific features of medical necessity make the concept particularly thorny. For example, part of the difficulty that physicians and patients experience within medical necessity decision-making processes and disagreements stems from the fact that medical necessity's terms of discourse fluctuate in relation to a diverse range of economic and social forces. Why, then, should researchers engaged with the question of medical necessity be surprised, not to mention "troubled," by their inability to locate a stable definition?[12] What assumptions give rise to the possibility that their results would or could be different? The answer resides somewhere between a failure to appeal to philosophy on the nature of contested concepts, the pragmatic difficulties inherent in using contestable concepts in policy debates, and a certain metaphysical assumption—perhaps a hope or an aspiration—that arises within language itself, where interlocutors come to assume or believe that rhetorical objects are more solid, fixed, and referential than they really are.

Despite the structural limitations of defining medical necessity in the abstract, attempts to do so can be found throughout both the scholarly and popular literature. Almost without exception, the consequence of these exercises is frustration and inconclusiveness. This dynamic reflects Glassman and colleagues' observation that "medical necessity means different things to patients, providers, and payers," even as it legally constitutes the "contractual basis between patients and insurers or health plans to provide medically necessary health care." Aside from the problem of tautology—cases in which the medically necessary is defined as what is deemed medically necessary—in practical terms the term is "used to determine whether a particular procedure or treatment should be provided."[13]

Medical Necessity as a Dynamic Concept

Having jettisoned the misguided idea that medical necessity can be defined in the abstract, we are left with the realization that medical necessity is a historical concept and product of mechanisms of change—conceptual, technological, economic, and political. To engage contemporary questions of medical necessity, which is the ultimate aim of this book, we must first consider, even in its broad strokes, not only medical necessity's development, but the roles played by key actors that have shaped that development over time. To tell this history requires attending to these actors' roles and vantage points.

Morreim notes that when "health insurance emerged in the 1930s and became a standard workplace benefit in the '40s and '50s, insurers nearly always deferred to physicians' judgments about what care a patient should have."[14] The concept of medical necessity became increasingly prominent during this time as a tool for securing payments for health care services. These arrangements, in turn, established a power dynamic for interpreting medical necessity. Early interpretive approaches were rooted in a tradition in which "insurers accepted the decisions of physicians about what was medically necessary without much question."[15] This period was one of relative physician sovereignty, where physicians were empowered to determine the contours of the discourse with little resistance from other actors. The ability and right for physicians to determine medical necessity in a relatively unfettered way was, in fact, a foundation of their professional standing and power.

In the 1960s, however, as health care costs exploded, health care insurers began to evoke the language of medical necessity to limit services.[16] The concept was a tool for overseeing and regulating providers and the services they were billing for. Over time, in a turn away from the 1950s' deference to physician determinations, insurers grew increasingly skeptical and started imposing restrictions. Rejections based on medical necessity in turn provoked government responses as new legal apparatuses began to arise.

By the 1970s, with the arrival of managed care, decision making had become subject to formal oversight by medical boards, insurance advisory bodies, and, eventually, government appeals panels. The arrival of these mechanisms led to blowback from patients and providers, and a brief flirtation with alternative concepts to circumvent medical necessity. Chief among these efforts was medical "appropriateness," which policymakers proposed as a translational term of art as part of ultimately unsuccessful Clinton-era health care reforms. Yet, this turn to appropriateness sent clinical and other decision makers down the same definitional rabbit hole as medical necessity had, especially since appropriateness was rendered dependent on defining additional terms such as "effective," "beneficial," and "judicious." As psychiatrist Daniel Knoepflmacher, a critic of the regulation of medical necessity, notes, each of these subterms had their own definitions as well.[17] Unable to resolve the broader question of defining medical necessity, medical appropriateness has continued to reappear from time to time, particularly in legal cases contesting insurance denials and the use of nebulous medical necessity criteria.

Medical necessity as we encounter it today is an outgrowth of dynamics established by managed care in the 1970s, tasked with making physicians "justify their previously unchallenged decisions."[18] Attempts to resolve the question in the abstract have provoked negative responses from various actors. But let us consider, more specifically, how individual actors and stakeholders in medical necessity debates have tended to engage the question.

Physicians

The changing place of physicians in American health care, whether perceived or real, is a critical context for understanding medical necessity's historical development. In 2017, Heather Lyu and colleagues published a much-discussed study based on an extensive physician survey that inquired into the prevalence of unnecessary care, and specifically "the extent of overutilization, as well as causes, solutions, and implications for health care."[19] According to the study, while overutilization is common, physicians themselves must be part of the solution, both in rethinking their assumptions and habits and in making their voices more prominent in devising solutions on both the practice and policy level. The findings suggested that physicians believed 20.6 percent of overall medical care, 22.0 percent of prescription medications, 24.9 percent of tests, and 11.1 percent of procedures to be unnecessary. The most common reasons given by respondents were "fear of malpractice," "patient pressure/request," and "difficulty accessing prior medical records." As a whole, the study finds that there is a problem of unnecessary care, which comes at a great cost to the American health system, with the potential to do great harm to patients. Just as important, however, though the report doesn't emphasize the point, is that physician perceptions drive the dynamics of the American health care system, whether those perceptions are correct or not.

Physicians often evoke this history as part of well-known (and seemingly increasingly common) narratives about the decline of their profession, which often amounts to a perceived loss of power and concern about burnout.[20] Whereas medical necessity originally strengthened physicians' place in health care utilization, ensuring that they received payments for their services, managed care used medical necessity to constrain them, limiting care or even refusing payment altogether.[21] The American Medical Association sees the history of medical necessity decision making under managed care not only as a threat to physician autonomy but one that has blurred the lines between clinical determinations and financial calculations. Specifically, it seeks to quarantine medical necessity from the corrosive effects of business. "Cost containment," it asserts, "has no place in medical necessity determinations."[22]

Some view these developments as having constituted a "radical shift in power" as medical necessity provided leverage that insurers could, and did, increasingly use against physicians.[23] Yet, the Foucauldian perspective reminds us that something more significant, subtle, and multifaceted is at work. Over time, the legitimating forces that enabled physicians' power to persist shifted amidst changes in the broader health care terrain, which became more tightly controlled. Physicians' determinations increasingly became entwined within a chorus of stakeholder voices that included patients, physicians, insurers and advisory boards, and a range of government and judicial entities. Medical necessity discourse began to both proliferate and fracture, morphing from an "obscure insurance term" to a "focus of national debates over who should make the coverage decisions, how those decisions should be made, and at what level of government."[24] To be sure, this focus on medical necessity may have been less of a central question that needed to be answered than a "convenient place for the armies to fight,"[25] as Foucault held that commonly evoked discourses often are.[26] The effect was, nonetheless, a contentious politics over medical necessity's definitional terms.

This suggests that the development of the American physician can be narrated, at least in part, through the politics of medical necessity. Despite growing concerns among physicians and their advocacy organizations about loss of autonomy, physicians remain the central actors in medical necessity decision making. Their training and socialization are therefore of great import. Considering that the Affordable Care Act (ACA) leaves previously existing medical necessity decision making intact, physicians' dilemmas remain essentially unchanged from the situation created by managed care, which applied greater oversight to physicians' judgments.

There is, of course, nothing sacred or infallible about physicians' judgments. They are, after all, just judgments—even if they are comparatively well informed. Noticing this fact upends the longstanding view of medical decision making, promoted most vociferously by physicians' advocacy groups who assert that a physicians' training suits them, and only them, for playing the role of a privileged spokesperson on behalf of medical need. If the AMA's position is to be accepted, physicians would act—at least in terms of how they are perceived—as relative sovereigns, even when they speak by way of medical appeals boards and other bodies. Of course, as one finds in the many physician lamentations posted across the internet, it often appears that payers ultimately determine medical necessity. And while this is, on its face, a disquieting thought, the inappropriateness of this fact is not obvious without further argument. Rather, it is through the politics of medical necessity itself that relative authority and credibility must be negotiated. While skepticism about payer motives is warranted, this does not mean that physicians are uniquely positioned to be the sole voice in medical necessity decision making. Indeed, from the perspective of persuasion, it must be acknowledged that physician authority has rarely been premised on an evidentiary base that can demonstrate that physicians are better at determining medical necessity than other bodies. This is the hard test for physicians.

Whether right or wrong, physicians are increasingly one voice among many in the contest over the meaning of medical necessity. Today, physicians' medical necessity determinations are mediated by shifting institutional, legal, moral, political, economic, and cultural dynamics. Interprofessional medical education is, to varying degrees, training physicians to view their role in decision-making processes as collaborative, with input not only from patients, but physicians' assistants, nurses and nurse practitioners, and even social workers. The infusion of health policy and management into medical education curricula is sending future physicians a message that they must learn how to navigate systems beyond clinical decision making if they are to successfully advocate for patients. Within this terrain, medical necessity is a function of more than physician consultations, suggesting that the modes of authority themselves may be shifting. While medical necessity determinations can no longer be understood as the sovereign control of physicians, neither can they be assumed to issue in an uncomplicated manner from the broader agreement of medical professionals. Certainly, to assume that medical necessity determinations are the simple purview of trained professionals is to take a too-narrow view of the cultural production of medical knowledge, and to accept an antiquated view of knowledge production—even in specialized domains. Medical necessity is increasingly a rhetoric with great cultural reach, about which many groups now feel capable of and willing to engage.

Of course, for those seeking a clear, reliable medical necessity standard, this proliferation of voices can be decentering. Hence the "cognitive confusion" some parents report when physicians do not agree on treatments for their children.[27] Parents' increasing empowerment, leading them to issue their own judgments, informed—correctly or incorrectly—by websites and apps and the onset of direct-to-consumer advertising, complicates this process. While this development amounts to a fundamental change in how Americans see medicine, this disassembling is of great significance for a legal system built around physicians' authority, especially in situations where physicians—and not the members of care teams who are consulted during the decision-making process—hold ultimate responsibility for outcomes.

The effects of these changes have been the source of "considerable litigation . . . prompted by patients challenging treatment denials based on medical necessity."[28] Yet in this area the law has evolved to empower health insurers against physicians as well as patients. Courts have determined—most notably in the 2000 decision *Pegram v. Herdrich*—that managed care organizations (MCOs) are shielded from responsibility for the medical necessity determinations made by physicians in their employ.[29] As the AMA laments, even as "MCOs across the country have taken control of medical decision making by blurring the definition of medical necessity—a clinical determination—with covered services—a business determination . . . [they] specifically disclaim any responsibility for medical decision making and seek to place all liability on physicians."[30]

Some physicians see a paradox insofar as they remain "a locus of accountability." As pediatrician and medical ethicist John Lantos notes,

> If things go badly, the doctors are to blame. If things are going to change, doctors have to be the leaders. In this role doctors, like insurance companies, become the embodiment of our belief that we are not helpless against the randomness of the world. If we don't like the way things turn out, we can hold the doctors responsible. We can punish them.[31]

This points to a bind in which physicians remain responsible even as their judgments are less able to operate unilaterally. As a result, physicians often encounter medical necessity as a hostile external force that confronts and calls into question their professional judgment.[32] In a different vernacular, their judgment is constrained.

There is, of course, good reason to consider the possibility that setting boundaries to physician authority must be part of the larger health care puzzle. Among the dimensions that play a role are increased specialization, changes in care philosophies that limit physicians' roles, changes in financing, and technological developments.[33] A number of financial strategies have been introduced to discipline physicians and change their behavior. For example, "capitated" plans set limits for care at a preset cost level. Under Alternative Payment Models championed by the Center for Medicare and Medicaid Innovation, physicians receive financial incentives to manage care efficiently while maintaining or improving outcomes.

We should expect all of this to bear on medical necessity decision making. The question is how and to what end. While patient outcomes remain the central concern of analysts who study these models, there is still a great deal of skepticism among various stakeholders. Though private interests and the increasing prevalence of for-profit medicine do not appear to be in and of themselves problems within these new payment models, it is nonetheless the case that there is widespread—even sometimes warranted—suspicion that such models are primarily driven by profit motives. The idea that the reduction of costs is, at base, good for expanded access and sustainability appear to arise as secondary matters within the politics of medical necessity. The very fact that medical necessity concerns power contributes to a palpable erosion of trust.

Some scholars see potential problems with such models, especially those that use capitation to reduce unnecessary and expensive health care services.[34] A study of the much-discussed Oregon Health System found that "most medical directors felt that capitation played a stronger role than the Prioritized List in determining how physicians approached patient care because most clinical decisions could not be made simply by referring to the list of covered condition-treatment pairs. . . . [Instead] the provision of covered benefits depended more on relatively unstructured physician decision making than on a structured medical necessity approach."[35] At the same time, the study found that financial incentives were more effective than medical necessity standards at promoting efficient individualized care. In other words, price controls and financial incentives appeared to constrain physicians' judgments more reliably than did fixed medical necessity schemas—so well in fact that Oregon "had to change its oversight function from preventing overuse to ensuring that Medicaid clients received needed items and services."[36] In the case of the Oregon program, narrow criteria swung so far in the opposite direction that the integrity of medical necessity decision making itself was called into question. This reminds us that physicians' roles in medical necessity decision making are intimately bound to structural constraints that "create the background against which [physicians] are forced to act."[37] Physicians do not make medical necessity judgments in a vacuum. They must advocate for their patients, particularly by participating in appeals and handling required documentation. As physicians are quick to note, most of this work is uncompensated.

It is also important to consider the possibility that some physicians mold medical necessity to satisfy financial interests, whether personal or institutional. The AMA's primary hedge against such possible abuses—a sort of inverse moral hazard—is the so-called "prudent physician" definition:

> Health care services or procedures that a prudent physician would provide to a patient for the purpose of preventing, diagnosing, or treating an illness, injury, disease, or its symptoms in a manner that is (a) in accordance with generally accepted standards of medical practice, (b) clinically appropriate in terms of type, frequency, extent, site, and duration, and (c) not primarily for the convenience of the patient, physician, or other health care provider.[38]

The "prudent physician" is the most commonly evoked standard as regards physician involvement with medical necessity. Yet, despite its ubiquity, the definition creates more questions than it solves and serves less as a solution than a fount from which disagreement flows. Not only is the notion of a "prudent physician" essentially contested (consider, for example, debates about physician assisted suicide and capital punishment[39]) but the terms by which prudence would have to be evaluated, laid out in (a), (b), and (c), give rise to a wide range of new questions. For example, the notions of "illness, injury, disease, or its symptoms" that the definition identifies as the ends of medical care are the subject of considerable disagreement. Since the "prudent physician" is central to the AMA definition, medical necessity tends to rise and fall with physicians' legitimacy.

This leaves us in a bind. Ascribing relatively unfettered agency to physicians is of course problematic. Research on variations in health care utilization has found that physicians' preferences—which still hold tremendous sway with patients—cannot be easily equated with expert medical consensus or even reasoned medical judgment. Certainly, physician judgment is to be respected, but showing respect is a different matter than ascribing it unchecked authority. John Wennberg's important research on variation suggests that medical necessity is often less a function of expertise than a result of cultural phenomena that produce multiple supply-side biases. Here, physicians with specialized expertise tend to influence one another such that what tends to be deemed medically necessary in one region could be vastly different—even medically unnecessary—in another.[40] This is compounded by evidence that many physicians hold racial, religious, and class biases that affect their decisions to declare something medically necessary for specific patients.[41]

It is important to notice how the racial biases of physicians interact with medical necessity. For example, a 2011 study that analyzed physicians' beliefs about the role of race in medical decision making found that "black physicians also stated that treating black patients more aggressively is necessary because of co-morbidities or increased risk for developing secondary conditions."[42] As one doctor put it, "In African Americans, hypertension [and] diabetes [are] more significant than that as compared to who is white or of a different race [because of] more severe problems with kidney control, kidney function." The authors also state that black physicians "viewed race as important for treatment decision making, while only four white physicians considered race medically relevant." This suggests that white physicians' biases might sometimes be rooted in their inattention to race, namely the belief that white and black patients face the same challenges and should, medically, be treated the same. While this belief could be interpreted as egalitarian, it ignores the population health and cultural obstacles that affect the health of African Americans, such as disproportionate diagnosis rates and the trauma of institutional racism.

The result is that what begins with a defense of individual physician judgments becomes increasingly observable as a broader social phenomenon, where various forms of social power—from the socialization of medical training to institutional and even regional biases—become an important part of understanding medical necessity decision making. As not only Foucault, but influential sociologists such as Paul Starr would no doubt agree, it is important to study physicians as embedded in, subjected to, and afforded subjectivity itself through broader orders of discourse and developmental histories.[43] To reduce physicians to clichés such as "doing what is best for their patients" is to overly simplify the complex psychology as well as power relations inherent in medicine. To extract from them a picture of autonomous, evidence-based, independent decision making is to misunderstand the role that stakeholding and identity play in American medicine.

Patients

These considerations lead to the obvious question of what role patients might play in medical necessity decision making. As with physicians, however, we cannot consider this question without placing patients in their own larger contexts. Like physicians, patients are certainly not, as most Americans would probably agree, sovereign voices within medical politics.

Consider, for example, the case of pharmaceuticals. Currently, the United States is the only nation to allow direct-to-consumer advertising for prescription drugs.[44] As critics of the pharmaceutical industry note, companies allocate large percentages of their total budgets to marketing, often eclipsing resources devoted to research and development.[45] While this is an important issue, this question intersects with the politics of medical necessity insofar as the circulation of television and other advertisements impact patients' thinking about medical necessity. Though we should not dismiss the potential benefits of patients educating themselves about their options, which many pharmaceutical companies claim advertising does, the educational value of such advertisements is highly dubious.[46]

At the same time, studies have cast doubt on the oft-repeated claim that patient preferences drive the use of medically unnecessary care.[47] This suggests a paradox, as patients are encouraged to pursue drugs that they themselves cannot purchase without a physician's approval, and that they are not trained to understand. While studies do suggest that people often know their health situation best,[48] there is good reason to be skeptical of patients' clinical understanding of their conditions, especially as concerns their license to declare a particular intervention medically necessary.[49] Medical rhetoric scholar Judy Z. Segal rightly criticizes skewing too far in the direction of patient expertise or self-diagnosis, noting that "equality rhetoric belongs to consumerist rhetoric and is a rhetoric of rights that may be inappropriate to questions of health and illness."[50] Accordingly, we must be critical of knowledge proliferating in the media, the effect of which is a situation in which patients calculate what they need from un-reliable sources or even stakeholder propaganda, both of which are some-times planted in physicians' offices. Physicians, in response, report feeling pressured to take their patients' assessments seriously, leading to efforts that cater to patient satisfaction, such as overprescribing.[51] What these problematic approaches have in common is that they are said to be driven to varying degrees by patient behaviors.

An effect of these dynamics is that patients are caught in, and no doubt confused and frustrated by, unstable discourses. The well-known Ameri-can advertising trope, "Ask your doctor if X is right for you?" plays upon such skepticism by suggesting that physicians may not be considering all options and that patients need to specifically recommend treatments and drugs to their physicians. It is also reasonable to consider that such adver-tisements may be a factor in the increasing fear on the part of physicians that is leading some to practice what is commonly known as "defensive medicine," a coinage marking situations in which physicians may uti-lize diagnostics, treatments, and drugs that may be marginally related to symptoms or even unnecessary—but do so to protect themselves from malpractice suits.[52]

John Lantos explains that "as a matter of legal and moral principle . . . doctors have dual loyalties," working for patients "but also, sometimes, for managed-care companies, corporations, drug companies, govern-ment agencies and others."[53] Within one of the most common discursive orders of contemporary medicine, this directly challenges claims to so-called patient-centeredness. Of course, depending on what is meant by patient-centeredness, some counterweight to patient conceptions of medi-cal necessity may be important. In some cases, the shift requires merely adjusting patient-physician communications.[54] In others, the relationship between patient preferences and health outcomes may be at odds. After all, despite attempts to link medical necessity with clinical trials and physician expertise, respecting culture requires understanding cultural diversity in clinical settings, as well as respecting "individuals' health beliefs, values, and behaviors."[55] Such work cannot be accomplished with one-size-fits-all rubrics or guidelines. Physician expertise must be paired with patient values, within the constraints of the systems within which both operate.

The National Academy of Medicine, formerly the Institute of Medicine, associates patient-centered care with "respecting and responding to patients' wants, needs, and preferences, so that they can make choices in their care that best fit their individual circumstances."[56] Within the broader politics of medical necessity, therefore, a true commitment to patient-centeredness requires a fundamental restructuring of decision-making authority and respect for patients' voices. There is a tension within a health care financing system that privileges needs over wants. Here, in other words, "Respecting and responding to" may not be the same as dispensing actual care in accordance with patients' wishes. More is at issue than simple choice.

New conceptual tools, or at least a fresh perspective, will be required if we are to avoid privileging physician, patient, and especially insurer determinations at the expense of more inclusive, broadly informed frameworks. Taking patient preference seriously, for example, Wennberg defines unnecessary surgery somewhat uniquely as "surgery on patients who do not want the operation."[57] For Wennberg, despite the contemporary deference to patient preferences, "informed consent" channels patients' preferences into physicians' preferences as patients tend to delegate and defer to physicians anyway. He counsels,

> Establishing a market where the utilization of preference-sensitive treatment is determined by patient demand will require a cultural change in the doctor-patient relationship. It will require replacing delegated decision-making with shared decision-making, and establishing informed patient choice as the standard of care for determining medical necessity.[58]

This suggests that fully-informed patients tend to be more conservative than their physicians, preferring management and "watchful waiting" to surgery. In Wennberg's view, this requires a move from "informed consent" toward what he calls "informed patient choice," which has more lately evolved into an approach known as "shared decision making." If informed consent turns out to reproduce physicians' choices and reinforce the perspective taken by their area of specialization and its professional organizations, informed patient choice and shared decision making seeks to disrupt physicians' preferences—the same ones that often yield unnecessary care—or at least decenter them. Such decentering comes by ensuring that multiple options are presented to patients, and often utilizes decision-making charts with graphics and decision trees.[59] These approaches aim to free medical necessity decision making from physician choice in a way that would likely decrease the frequency of aggressive medical interventions, reducing utilization as well as costs without negatively affecting morbidity or mortality. The ultimate goal of these approaches is not only to alter existing power relations, but to improve outcomes. The reaction that physicians often have to such suggestions reminds us that the decentralization of patient care requires a reconfiguration not only of medical power, but clinicians' identities.

Patients are often evoked within the politics of medical necessity as part of a larger discourse of responsibility. This makes sense since, as we know, medical necessity promises to maintain the distinction, for example, between physical therapy and routine exercise, or psychotherapy, psychiatry, and the "normal" human condition. But what underlies these distinctions? These discourses—particularly as they appear with socially-laden themes such as diet, exercise, and sexuality—emphasize medical necessity's ability to hedge moral hazard stemming from the supposedly irresponsible actions of individuals that, in turn, could threaten the fiscal sustainability of systems and insurance arrangements. This image of health care "does not start from what people want but from what they need,"[60] while establishing a moral distinction between society's responsibilities to the different camps, based on the origin of their needs.

Payers

To state the obvious, insurance company interests are different from those of physicians and patients. At the same time, they participate in the same epistemic project of distinguishing the medical from the contrasting concepts we have explored. Of course, there is good reason for doing this from the perspective of the politics of medicine. After all, some medical necessity definitions transcend the medical as it is typically construed, such as those that consider the traditional view of medicine to lack the tools required to adequately address health on the population level, where the social determinants of health are the focus. Ireys and colleagues advocate an approach focused on allowing patients "to achieve or maintain sufficient functional capacity to perform age-appropriate or developmentally appropriate daily activities."[61] This requires that many considerations be made "beyond 'medical evidence.'"[62]

A linguistic paradox arises from a conceptualization of medical necessity that exceeds the rhetorical promise of the medical in order to meet patients' health needs. This dynamic turns out to be true of the medical as well as the rhetoric of necessity generally, suggesting a need for rethinking not only necessity, but its modifier "medical."[63] These proposals find value in the rhetoric of necessity but would rethink the predicate—"health necessity," "treatment necessity," or "clinical necessity"—to detach care from its thin and contested medical grounding. Within the context of financial considerations, we should expect that companies will seek to exploit these rhetorical distinctions.

Peter Conrad and Valerie Leiter note that, "By restricting access to medical solutions in the name of medical necessity, insurers attempt to limit individuals' claims that they are suffering from illnesses rather than everyday life."[64] The more critical point is that these companies have a direct financial stake in employing the most restrictive conception of medical necessity possible. As part of this language game, a delineated view of the medical justifies a narrow scope of financial responsibility, while ignoring broader contours of health. Just as libertarian critics of medical necessity are concerned about the moral hazard that expansive notions of medical necessity might yield on the side of patients, insurance companies would be inversely affected by such an expansion as restrictive conceptions of medical necessity could yield financial rewards.

Medical necessity's definitional instability opens important spaces for argument on the part of critics of the American insurance industry who suspect that medically necessary treatments are being excluded for financial instead of medical reasons. In the United States, such considerations have received legal sanction. In *Pegram*, for example, the Supreme Court argued that, "no [health maintenance organization] could survive without some incentive connecting physician reward with treatment rationing."[65]

Rationing, the court found, is part of medical decision making undertaken within the kind of cost containment models that govern managed care. Given the importance of setting priorities in health care utilization through medical necessity determinations, the only question that remains concerns the drawing of definitional lines to govern such prioritization. Politically, the specter of rationing is fueled in part by concerns about how qualitative distinctions are made within medical necessity debates. Ireys and colleagues explain this as follows:

> Another purpose for a clear definition of medical necessity is to distinguish it from "rationing." By definition, rationing means "to distribute equitably." It implies the withholding of treatment on the basis of both cost and outcome considerations. Rationing is a deliberate, if uncomfortable, decision to protect resources for the group as a whole at the expense of individual needs. Decisions about rationing must balance individual and group needs in light of expected costs. In contrast, decisions on medical necessity must be based on an individual's medical, health, and family situation, and not on cost.[66]

Though discussions about rationing in American politics have tended to devolve into questions of who does and who does not advocate rationing, the more important question is how to do so fairly and transparently. Instead of labeling rationing, queuing, and triaging as a matter of ideology, it is more accurate and useful to view it as a fact of all health care decision making.

At the same time, medical necessity decision making is only useful insofar as certain analytic categories remain distinct and stable. The intermingling of facts and values make such pretenses to analytic stability difficult to maintain. The *Pegram* decision, for example, also held that coverage determinations and treatment decisions were essentially indistinguishable, making it hard to identify the origins of constraints on medical necessity. The court noted,

> Although coverage for many conditions will be clear and various treatment options will be indisputably compensable, physicians still must decide what to do in particular cases. The issue may be, say, whether one treatment option is so superior to another under

the circumstances, and needed so promptly, that a decision to proceed with it would meet the medical necessity requirement that conditions the HMO's obligation to provide or pay for that particular procedure at that time in that case.

Here again, *Pegram* acknowledges rationing's centrality to the very idea of managed care. Yet, the court also identifies physicians as the central reason why such measures are necessary, noting that "HMOs came into being because some groups of physicians consistently provided more aggressive treatment than others in similar circumstances, with results not perceived as justified by the marginal expense and risk associated with intervention." Essentially declaring moral hazard to be inevitable within such systems, the court noted that "it would be so easy to allege, and to find, an economic influence when sparing care did not lead to a well patient, that any such standard in practice would allow a factfinder to convert an HMO into a guarantor of recovery."[67] The result is a restructuring of priorities, as scholars have noted as well.[68]

The consensus that medical necessity decision making can consider cost is therefore both well established and legally protected, at least for those plans falling under the jurisdiction of the Employment and Retirement Income Security Act of 1974 (ERISA) which regulates large employer markets and federal insurance programs. The strongest reading of *Pegram* is that the case amounts to a defense of managed care itself. The court notes, for example, that *Pegram*'s "remedy in effect would be nothing less than elimination of the for-profit HMO" and possibly "even more than that." As such, the court not only fails to help with the question of defining medical necessity, but introduces financial consideration into the calculus.

Appealing Medical Necessity Determinations

As is the case with all definitional questions, authority matters. The Foucauldian framework reminds us that authority is not a simple matter of an individual empowered to decide, but is best grasped as a function of a complex series of networks through which power flows. This raises an important question: if physicians are increasingly unable to persuade health insurance providers or their appeals committees that care is necessary, who is positioned to advocate for patients? Certainly not, in the current system, patients themselves. One answer is lawyers. As the Pennsylvania Health Law Project explains,

> [if a physician has] prescribed something for your patient which you believe is indicated, and the insurance issues a denial, the best way to help your patient is to write an excellent letter of medical necessity and to participate in the fair hearing. The patient does not need a lawyer, but does need the physician's help, including clear medical record notes documenting the need.[69]

If physicians feel that they are unable to represent their patients adequately, however, the organization is available for legal representation. Rather than reading medical necessity as a dual medical and legal question, as the Foucauldian might, the Pennsylvania Health Law Project evacuates the concept of its medical content and declares that "medical necessity is a legal, not a medical, definition." If this is true, then should we evaluate medical necessity decision making in a similar way as legal interpretation? And, if so, does the literature on legal rhetoric and interpretation apply?

The American health care system, as I have noted, is an often-disjointed admixture of private and public health care systems, with various roles of oversight performed by states and the federal government. Physicians, patients, and payers are located within systems of internal and external appeals that possess the force of law. Each of these layers provides not only important modes of recourse and rights for the various actors involved— especially in the form of counterweights for patients against payers—but serves as a means of overturning, questioning, and changing how the actors themselves approach medical necessity.[70]

In general, medical necessity appeals are written requests to review and change an adverse determination made by an insurance provider. Though most states mandate formal appeals processes, albeit with significant variation from state to state, the ACA established a patient right for the appeal of insurance decisions and put forth standards for internal and external reviews.[71] Perhaps most important, the bill mandated procedures in the event that a state's appeals processes do not meet federal consumer protection standards, funneling those cases into a federally-administered external review process carried out by a federally accredited Independent Review Organization or an HHS-led external review, conducted at no cost to insurers.[72]

Despite the ACA's advances in this area, establishing effective oversight remains a challenge. This is for the predictable reason that the various participants in these decision-making processes, even those tasked with overseeing appeals and carrying out regulatory oversight, often disagree on the meanings of key terms. Such disagreement makes applying principles in a systematic manner difficult and reaching consensus even more so.

This insight points to at least two different possibilities. First, it suggests that there is little hope of settling medical necessity disagreements at the regulatory level. The best one can hope for is a qualitatively different determination, but one that carries the force of law or at least the persuasive ability to secure care for patients. Indeed, if regulators and medical directors can't agree on an abstract definition of these terms, how could they be expected to agree on particular judgments? The difference appears to concern which standards are operationalized within legal and policy domains.

Second, there may be even more contention at the regulatory level than among medical professionals. On the surface, this is a disquieting possibility, since regulatory schemas promise to play a positive role in settling disputes. Yet, from a slightly different vantage point, this contention could turn out to be good for patients since regulators may be more willing to construe medical necessity broadly, as they are not beholden to any one specific interest. They could value, above all, what they construe to be in the interest of patients, or perceived public, or some other value set. The concern, of course, would be discriminatory practices on the part of regulators. In response, it could be that a federally-regulated appeals process might ensure that any unevenness on the state level would be subjected to systematic oversight. But, here again, "layering a uniform review and appeals system atop such a variable decision-making process may, at the end of the day, make access to medical care less—rather than more—consistent."[73] As one commentator noted some years ago, if medical necessity decision making is often inconsistent, then it is also true that "consistency is equally challenging in reviews of medical necessity."[74]

The ACA did address these areas of concern. Section 2719 requires that health care providers establish "effective" appeals processes for both "coverage determinations and claims."[75] As part of these requirements, plans must maintain an internal appeals process, and

> provide notice to enrollees, in a culturally and linguistically appropriate manner, of available internal and external appeals processes,

and the availability of any applicable office of health insurance consumer assistance or ombudsman . . . to assist such enrollees with the appeals processes.

Enrollees must be allowed to review their files and participate in the appeals process while receiving "continued coverage pending the outcome of the appeals process." Finally, providers must have in place external review processes that meet standards established by the National Association of Insurance Commissioners' Uniform External Review Model Act. In other words, these medical necessity appeals are governed by an altogether different interpretive regulatory schema.

Given the variability present in efforts to govern medical necessity decision making at the level of physician judgment and payer approval, the qualitative nature of the appeals processes over which HHS has oversight are key. Specifically, the HHS secretary is tasked with establishing appeals processes that will "enable individuals to appeal a determination under this section; [and support] procedures to protect against waste, fraud, and abuse."[76] Only if HHS is able to protect the integrity of the decision-making processes that enable patients to access benefits via medical necessity determinations will the ACA effectively connect its benefits provisions to the delivery of actual medical care. But the politics required to do so—especially given the heated rhetoric of "death panels" initiated by ACA opponents during the early days of the bill's implementation—make such efforts politically challenging.[77] Yet, it is also true that inhospitable political moments usually wane, as when, in October 2015, with little fanfare, the death panel debate gave way as billable end-of-life planning was authorized by Medicare.[78]

The quality of medical necessity determinations made on appeal depends on the interests embedded within them, as well as integrity of the processes through which appeals are undertaken. While internal appeals administered by insurance providers are often viewed with skepticism because of the self-interestedness of stakeholders, external appeals are intended to instill confidence in medical necessity decision making precisely because they are external. This confidence in external review gestures toward the possibility of certain institutions making necessity determinations that are, in a sense, "real," or at least uncorrupted by interests adverse to those of patients.

As internal appeals often lack the perception of objectivity due to potential conflict of interest, the authority and hope of external appeals processes rests on a perception of disinterestedness that promises to resist potentially corrupt internal processes, especially profit-seeking behaviors under the guise of medical decisions. These processes, regulated by the state and governed by professional norms, promise to hedge against health insurance provider medical necessity determinations. The question is what keeps these appeals processes from amounting to the mere shifting of authority—what rhetoric scholars call "ethos"—while still potentially failing to meet patients' needs, whether real or perceived.

It is important to take note of the theoretical assumptions built into the internal-external dichotomy, particularly as the very idea of externality is believed to produce a more accurate and fair conception of medical necessity.[79] A first assumption concerns the persuasive effects of externality—the great hope of external appeals. It is important to note that any persuasiveness externality might have would seem to issue from the perceived disinterestedness of bodies empowered to decide, or perhaps the distance such people might have from key stakeholders. A second, somewhat stronger position holds that external reviewers possess formal protections against the conflicts of interest that cast internal reviews with doubt. Such external reviewers are supposed to be placed in such a way as to avoid the kind of conflicts of interest that undermine the judgments of other actors.

Such boundary drawing, however, depends on a theory of knowledge that is institutionally bound, where language can be contained neatly as either clinical or economic. For example, if neoliberal perspectives that privatize responsibility for health outcomes flow freely between internal and external bodies, then externality loses some or even all of its appeal. If patients' rights or physicians' judgments are afforded high degrees of legitimacy even when larger institutions may push back, then such external bodies may play an important role. On the other hand, if neoliberal concepts such as efficiency, costs and benefits, and return on investment are part of the consideration, then the move from internal to external decision making secures little more than a perception. What is most important to acknowledge is that there is nothing about externality itself that ensures that medical necessity determination will be perceived as legitimate.

It is in this light that we must assess the ACA's promise to guarantee the integrity of medical necessity decision making by mandating that independent review organizations are subject to the oversight of accreditors such as the Utilization Review Accreditation Commission (URAC).

URAC seeks to cultivate a reputation of objectivity by declaring independence from industry stakeholders and maintaining a diverse board of directors. They are intended to ensure that external reviewers "are utilizing the most appropriate clinical and administrative procedures."[80] With this mandate, the ACA puts great weight on the abstract ideas of externality and independence. This suggests that precisely because they are perceived as impartial, groups charged with enforcing the ACA's antidiscrimination provisions, as well as the pursuit of ethical and efficacious health care more generally, must remain attuned to the unstated normative dimensions of these bodies' decision-making processes.

Insofar as medical necessity is constrained by benefits, utilization management, or "techniques used by health insurers to manage the use of covered benefits in the case of individual patients,"[81] is also unlikely to resolve the question of medical necessity. Utilization management is, after all, largely a function of medical necessity determinations made in relation to specific patients with specific conditions who, in their particularity, cannot be easily or ethically subsumed under general rules.

Perhaps the biggest mistake one could make in approaching appeals is assuming that appeals processes might mitigate or somehow evade the effects of social power. The existence of even objective or disinterested appeals does not guarantee that independent reviews are not encumbered by problematic conceptions of the body, such as health, wellness, and ability. As legal scholar Vernellia Randall notes, "these attempts to have the physician become the gatekeeper to medical care will ultimately change the entire structure of the American health care system and not necessarily for the better. The least articulate, least educated, least financially well-off person will have the most limits imposed by cost containment efforts."[82] As we'll see in chapter 4, one's degree of respect for mental health diagnoses and criteria can have important effects on medical necessity decision making.

The prominent health policy scholar and lawyer Sara Rosenbaum notes, "certain types of medical necessity decisions involve purely legal interpretations related to the content of coverage," while "appealable cases are those that rest on factual questions to be resolved by a decision maker."[83] This suggests that it is the quality of the decision that is most important, not the mere existence of appeals. This is not to say that external appeals are inherently suspect—they are for obvious reasons more attractive than internal appeals. It is to say, instead, that the perception that they operate outside of existing orders of power/knowledge is worth considering. It would be a mistake to assume that externality in and of itself can produce a more just or otherwise better medical necessity decision-making process. Indeed, considering externality's persuasive dimensions and promise of escaping bias and the interests of stakeholders, externality may even have the opposite effect, as ordinarily critical participants in medical necessity decision-making processes assume that all is well.

Insofar as all institutions are dependent upon concepts, medical necessity might be said to be a functionally necessary, or at least useful, evil. We shall explore the possibility of dispensing with it altogether, or conceding to its policy permanence, in the book's conclusion. For now it must suffice to note that the medical necessity with which we appear stuck for the moment is no mere concept among concepts, but one with specific entailments, a unique history, and one that plays a key role in shaping the current American health care system. Understanding its ambiguity and definitional contours is therefore of critical importance.

At the same time, it is not enough to understand medical necessity's conceptual contours; we must situate the concept's meaning within the stakeholding interests, locations, and the various actors—patients, payers, physicians, and appeals processes—that play key roles in definitional negotiations. Ultimately, this chapter does not offer a solution for resolving the political tensions with which medical necessity presents us. Rather, it positions us to see past some of the easier or more intuitive options, such as deferring to physicians or patients, so that we can begin to wrestle with some of medical necessity's thornier conceptual questions.

This analysis raises questions about the level of variability implicit in medical decision making—particularly as this variability relates to the languages through which we codify, catalog, and even casually speak about medical need. It also underscores the questions of power that are always present within medical necessity decision making. With this in mind, a critical next step is to look more closely at the formal codification systems through which medical necessity is systematized—systems that track disease, promote wellness, and, especially in the United States, determine payment.

2

In the Archive

Coding for Necessity and the Necessity of Coding

The previous chapter established that medical necessity must be approached as a contextual and political question. Rhetorically, however, it appears not as contextual or political, but as a fixed object of reference, which gives rise to the central question with which this book is concerned. The divide between medical necessity's reality and its rhetorical situation poses more than just an interpretive problem; it opens the way for a new set of questions. Medical necessity's political valence stems precisely from the fact that it resists a stable, definitional metaphysics and is therefore inherently contestable. To grasp medical necessity as a discursive production arising out of health care politics, we must concern ourselves with the proliferation of the language through which medical necessity appears—from casual small talk to formal documents such as coding schemes and policy guidelines.

My analysis is informed by Jacques Derrida's notion of the archive. According to Derrida, the archive must be considered in relation to its etymological relationship with the Greek *archein*, a word that signifies beginning as well as ruling.[1] According to Derrida, the person who controls the archive—the *archon*—is empowered to shape epistemic fields, from the writing of contextual histories to patient record narratives to what is and what is not considered necessary. At the same time, managing the archive requires the stabilization of meanings,—despite the fact that they are riddled by instability and tentativeness. It is here that the Derridean approach requires specifically rhetorical analysis, as a pretense to stopping movement within shifting semantic chains is both constitutive of coding's importance to contemporary health care and one of its central problems.[2] The archon is helpless to control the interpretation of discourses flowing within his holdings, but clings to appearances of sovereign power nonetheless.

This chapter's turn to the archive draws on Foucault's work on the "clinic"—the institution that can be said to historically have given rise to the medical archive.[3] This chapter is an investigation of two spaces—the clinic and the archive, understood expansively, even metaphorically—that play critical roles in negotiating medical rhetoric and epistemology. The establishment of this archive raises a particular set of concerns that informs both the politics of medical necessity and its relation to medical coding, record keeping, and other techniques through which medical necessity is deposited, recorded, stored, accessed, stabilized, and utilized. The increasingly central role that coding plays in American medicine recognizes that medical perception—the event through which this archival process is first initiated—must be translated into a medical discourse which, in turn, shapes the material investments and interventions that occur in medical situations.[4] Though the role of medical perception is clear in scholarship produced by Foucault and his followers over recent years, this focus must be directed to understanding how coding and increasingly stringent demands of record keeping are changing in relation to rapid developments in health care reform. One indication is the rise of coding and billing as a career trajectory, a particularly energetic area of employment growth in the United States. At the same time, the arrival of coding regimes such as the ICD-10 (the tenth edition of the International Classification of Diseases, Injuries, and Causes of Death), "meaningful use" standards for electronic medical records, and the ACA's "essential benefits" provisions suggest that a critical reading of medical necessity requires rethinking the archive.

Medical coding illustrates the depth of the institutional and discursive contexts in which medical necessity arises and operates. It also marks the precise moment where medical decision making is standardized in clinical, and even economic, contexts. While there has been a recent proliferation of the breadth of medical conditions within coding regimes, there has also been a deepening of the significance of medical coding more generally as payment systems tighten and public monies become increasingly attached to value-based outcomes. Taken together, these dual movements of breadth and depth position medical coding formidably within the broader politics of medical necessity and suggest a development of great relevance to those interested in grasping medical necessity as a political phenomenon.

Placing the politics of medical necessity in relation to the archive requires examining not only what is in the archive and what is not, but what gets released to whom, who controls the terms by which medical necessity discourse is ordered and given value, and who gets to decide what becomes official medical knowledge. The story of the medical necessity archive therefore mirrors—on the level of writing, construed broadly—the rise of medical necessity itself: from its most common origins in a physician's voice to the various actors in medical necessity's broader politics as health care becomes both more technically sophisticated and expensive. Predictably, the internet contributed to the expansion of the medical archive, with social media such as #MedicalNecessity on Twitter serving as a real-time compendium of medical necessity claims, outrage, and disagreement. Reading the medical necessity archive for the values that are inscribed there helps us to grasp it as a repository of power relations within medical discourse.

Compared to how we find it today, the medical necessity archive was decentralized in medicine's quainter days, when smaller private physician practices proliferated and the strings of oversight and utilization review were looser. Historically, we can mark the time when centralization began to intensify with the arrival of managed care which, in a sense, arose to address medical necessity itself. Since that period, though insurgent voices persist, the medical necessity archive has increasingly become the purview of large institutions, both public and private, paralleling the arrival of new layers of regulatory oversight as medicine has advanced and become more expensive. At the center of these developments stands a growing list of managerial experts and professional stakeholders, each of whom weighs in on the meaning of necessity, seeking to structure the labyrinthine world of medical coding in which illnesses and conditions get formalized into a recognizable discourse. Epistemic shifts in medicine have been met by a proliferation of voices.

Actors in the Archive

As I noted in the introduction and explored in depth in chapter 1, most patients become aware of medical necessity when a treatment that they or their physician deems necessary is rejected. This makes sense since, as philosophers (following Wittgenstein) know, language only presents itself as language when one is forced to confront it as such. Only at that point must patients and advocates navigate what Patricia Aalseth calls the "rejection puzzle."[5] Rejection, however, does not merely lead to clarity, but creates a need for further codes. Here, coding is cast as a chain of references, with codes justified by additional codes, eluding a center. Taken at its most basic level, medical necessity is an interpolative claim made with reference to a diagnosis, *marked* by a code. Denials are issued when a procedure's necessity is contested in light of a diagnosis. This underscores the extent to which judgment and rhetorical framing stand alongside reason and evidence, as politics arises in the spaces between.

The rhetoric commonly deployed to discuss medical coding reveals a number of important epistemic distinctions that give rise to such a politics. Aalseth, a coding expert, notes, "If you receive a denial notice from the payer that the procedure was 'not medically necessary' it means that your payer does not think the procedure or test was justified for the diagnosis given."[6] But—leaving aside the slippage from logical necessity to a rhetoric of justification—this interpretive claim is clearly not true. Rather, the political reading moves medical necessity claims to the level of just that: a claim. Where Aalseth seems to assume good faith (conflating what the payer "thinks" with what the payer "claims"), a political reading begins with skepticism, casting medical necessity claims as speech acts in need of context to assess their persuasive force. Accordingly, patient inquiries and physician pushback are often successful at reversing denials, underscoring the extent to which the objectivity of denials is far more subjective and contestable than claims reveal. When one pushes on this objectivity, it often falls apart.

Given the possibility of denials, physicians often establish multiple lines of defense. For example, providers who are concerned that payers will reject claims routinely have their patients sign Advance Beneficiary Notices (ABN) in which patients assume financial responsibility for rejected claims. Payers may also "downcode" claims, rejecting higher order (and often costlier) treatments, replacing them with lower order codes, combating what they perceive to be a tendency on the part of physicians and their staffs to "upcode." The question, as the AMA notes, is whether such alterations are medically justified.[7] This view misses the nature of coding itself, which travels in grays, not blacks and whites. Coding does not simply *prove* medical necessity through its ability to establish, through the rhetorical practices, that needs are real. Coding persuades. Obviously, the requirement that clinicians attend to this persuasive dimension produces feedback loops in which physicians must consider how care is coded even as they observe conditions and generate treatment options. Of even more concern is the possibility that physicians might begin to *see* options through the filter of coding, even to a point where coding comes to supplant observation itself, preceding and structuring observation.

It is worth breaking down the process. First, a physician examines a patient and records what he or she sees. What he or she sees, in turn, is necessarily shaped by the patient's particular goals, which are themselves the culmination of a process in which advertising and other social inputs undoubtedly play a role. Here, as Foucault notes, "The clinical gaze has the paradoxical ability to *hear a language* as soon as it *perceives a spectacle.*"[8] Refracting these observations through patient and family histories as well as other contexts, the physician then makes a diagnosis and recommends a course of action. However, we have not yet entered into the domain of medical coding which (considering the rules, legal and otherwise, that govern its current state) proceeds from physicians' observations and recodes them in the language of the controlling texts. Clinicians and their staffs are of course expected to master these texts, perhaps unreasonably. Such mastery is not a one-time commitment, moreover, but requires continuing education, certification and recertification, and vigilance.

Assuming such mastery is attainable, judgment serves as the basis of the codification process. This movement from seeing to judgment, then judgment to coding, does not carry force of its own, but must be sanctioned by insurance providers who either preauthorize medical services or review the medical necessity of services already rendered. They must locate themselves within a preestablished discourse. This theme of seeing, connected to the language through which patients' situations are understood, is threaded throughout critical literature in medicine. Luhrmann notes, with regard to the divide between biomedical and psychodynamic theoretical frameworks, that "what one learns to do affects the way one sees."[9] A similar insight underpins the steadily increasing respect for and acknowledge of the value in the medical humanities, including the role that art plays in training students[10] and the important role that interdisciplinarity has to play in ensuring that medical research is positioned to respond to changes in medicine, especially as "patient-centeredness" and "innovation" in health systems become real commitments, with real institutional support, beyond sloganeering.[11]

This turn toward a humanistic approach reminds us that medical records can only be systematized through an act of translation. This is no small task, not only because coding language itself is often inscrutable, but because the language to be translated is often a compilation of complicated and disjointed scribbles jotted down by physicians and other clinicians. This need for translation puts considerable pressure on office staff, from scribes to billers and office managers—one need only talk with these professionals to hear the frustration that those tasked with coding often experience, even in a world in which electronic medical records are slowly ironing out kinks.

Contemporary developments have inserted patients into the process as well, especially with the proposal that patients play a role in editing and maintaining their own health records.[12] This point underscores a tension inherent in working with codes for establishing medical necessity as a matter of professional training and privilege, on the one hand, and patient experience and self-advocacy, on the other. Medical coding is the outcome of a process through which records are made legible to insurers, appeals boards, and other actors in health care procurement and delivery. As one would expect, coding regimes are mostly unknown to the very patients to whom they refer, and who often experience medical necessity as a kind of interpellation, as seemingly routine medical treatment requires that one be subsumed in an external discourse. As such, we must be concerned with the discursive processes through which this conversion occurs as well as the experience of encountering them.

Key Documents

Before examining specific processes, we must first consider the archive as a whole to understand its conceptual foundation. A striking feature of the medical necessity archive is the sheer volume of documents that comprise its holding; it is not only large, but continually expanding and evolving. This is true for a number of reasons. First, as new technologies become available, medical expectations rise and options proliferate.[13] The need for new codes, moreover, is not a function of a simple outgrowth of technology, but a function of multiple factors, from efforts to deliver better and more efficient care to fraud prevention and regulatory oversight. All of this arises under the specter of rising costs, which coding schemes promise to rein in. Ironically, the expansion of coding schemes in the name of efficiency creates the need for larger staffs to perform new roles.[14] The need to define medical necessity is accompanied by efforts vis-à-vis medical coding to discipline and distinguish the necessary from the unnecessary.

The ICD, first developed in 1949 by the Centers for Medicare and Medicaid Services and the National Center for Health Statistics, remains the centerpiece of the politics of medical coding and the "bible" of medical necessity. The ICD is an internationally recognized diagnostic tool maintained and published by the World Health Organization (WHO), currently available in forty-three languages. As WHO explains, the ICD, now in its eleventh revision, is used to track population-level health data, especially the incidence and prevalence of diseases, as well as by individual medical practitioners and their office managers and coders. On the system level, the ICD is also widely used as a tool for standardizing reimbursement and allocating health care resources.[15]

It is important to note that the updating process itself is part of the proliferation and refinement of medical necessity discourse, as the ICD-10 moved from –three to five character codes in the ICD-9 to –three to seven character codes in the ICD-10, and from about 13,000 codes in the ICD-9 to about 68,000 in ICD-10.[16] An examination of the medical necessity archive requires careful consideration not only of specifics contained with the ICD, but the idea of the ICD itself, the very existence of which tells us something important about the administration of modern health care. Such an examination also requires understanding the purpose of ancillary texts, including the politics of their production and complicating factors such as controversies and conflicts of interest. This is more radical than it might at first seem. As theorist Terry Eagleton argues:

> The language of a legal document or scientific textbook may impress or even intimidate us because we do not see how the language got there in the first place. . . . Part of the power of such texts thus lies in their suppression of what might be called their modes of production, how they got to be what they are; in this sense, they have a curious resemblance to the life of the human ego, which thrives by repressing the process of its own making.[17]

Each text has its own history. At the same time, because of the nature of medical necessity decision making, no one text is determinate or able to control the writing of broader discursive boundaries. As we should expect, the relationships of power/knowledge that govern medical necessity decision making as it relates to coding are always shifting and subject to challenges.

While the ICD is a standard, federally required health diagnostic tool for classifying inpatient services, the AMA's Current Procedural Terminology (CPT) manual, first introduced in 1966, contains codes, descriptions, and guidelines to describe office and outpatient procedures and services performed by health care providers. Unlike ICD, which is publicly available, CPT is a copyrighted tool that is also the centerpiece of CMS's Healthcare Common Procedure Coding System (HCPCS). In addition, where the ICD is concerned with diagnoses, CPT codes identify billable services. Taken generally, the HCPCS aims to provide consistency in referring to services and products utilized in the contexts of healthcare. Since the introduction of the Health Insurance Portability and Accountability Act of 1996 (HIPAA), use of HCPCS has become mandatory for all health practitioners in the United States, not only to ensure privacy of records, but to promote consistency (and reduced variation, within practices as well as geographically) across various levels of care.

Specialized professional organizations have developed coding schemes of their own to address more specific needs. Included in this category is the International Classification of Functioning, Disability and Health (ICF) and Code on Dental Procedures and Nomenclature (CDT). While many of these specialized coding schemas occupy distinct epistemic territories, there are some notable areas in which different texts, backed and promoted by their professional interests and constituencies, jockey for the ability to control the order of discourse. Perhaps the most controversial and widely discussed of these texts is the *Diagnostic and Statistical Manual* (DSM) of the American Psychiatric Association, the primary mechanism for coding psychiatric assessment and diagnosis, which serves as a key tool for identifying treatment strategies and billing insurance accordingly. Unlike the ICD, which is free and readily available on the internet and contains mental health coding schemes that are not radically different from the DSM, the DSM is a major source of revenue for the American Psychiatric Association (APA). The profitability of the DSM has cast doubt in the minds of some practitioners about whether it is best regarded as an important coding resource or as a financing mechanism. Psychiatrist Gary Greenberg, a prominent critic of the medicalization of psychiatry, explains, "When it was released in 1952, the DSM's nomenclature imposed some order on the professional landscape. As insurance payments came to play an increasing role in the medical marketplace, those new diagnoses proved useful, especially to private-practice doctors."[18] Adding to the skepticism that grips Greenberg and others is the fact that more than half of the board members tasked with overseeing the DSM revision process are employed by pharmaceutical companies.[19]

To grasp the discourse of medical necessity is to a large extent to master these texts. Because these texts have been naturalized into American health care, however, the unique role codification plays often goes unnoticed. When this process is uncovered, as I have noted, it is usually the result of conflict, as when one is denied authorization for a medical service. At this point, operating in multiple discursive spaces, one simultaneously encounters a medical and financial space. Yet, given the level of particularity associated with the concept of medical necessity, it is revealing that medical coding, and coding for medical necessity in particular, is concerned with—as the authors of one textbook put it—"abstracting from medical records."[20] Medical records, in this view, are understood to be highly dependable and translatable documents in need of further systematization.

A final critical component of medical coding centers on evaluation and management coding (E&M), which is a three-tier process in which the patient's history is reviewed, an exam is performed, and medical decisions are made. A critical part of patient histories is the "chief complaint," which "consists of the patient's statement describing symptoms, problems, and other factors that brought him or her to seek medical care." Evoking a distinction between objective and subjective aspects of medical classification, Kelly-Farwell and Favreau deem this state the "*subjective* part of the visit" since it is "usually in the patient's or family members' own words."[21] The chief complaint is followed by a review of the patient's history recorded in relation to their complaint, a review of their body systems (usually derived from a patient questionnaire), and a personal and family history. Notice how this part of the visit is considered objective insofar as it does not include patient perspective. Physicians' perspectives, findings from exams, and personal and family history are considered objective by default.

The growing amount of paperwork required in contemporary American medicine is, of course, a common complaint among clinicians. Social scientists have also taken note. Luhrmann, for example, notes,

> [as] hospitalization goes on, more and more pages are added: nursing notes, psychiatrists' notes, notes from the occupational

therapist and the social worker and so forth. Each subsequent admission adds more paper. Soon the patient's chart—the folder with his name on it—bulges out to one inch, then to three . . .[22]

Luhrmann's account, written in 2000, may seem somewhat quaint in a contemporary moment when electronic medical records have replaced the folders she describes. Nor is the recognition that data collected in clinical situations is growing necessarily a commentary on medical necessity. For present purposes, however, it suffices to note only that the proliferation of paperwork—whether digital or not—creates the discursive raw material from which medical necessity is extracted and rhetorically produced.

From the perspective of most clinicians and their staffs, of course, the less coding from these documents the better. The expanded set of codes under ICD-10 has evoked a particularly loud chorus of concerns from physicians, even as many seem to have accepted that ICD-9, with which they were familiar, had outlived its usefulness. What is clear is that most physicians trust their own judgment and resist preestablished discursive regimes that constrain that judgment—which is one reason why some are advocating new systems of medical care located outside of insurance arrangements, such as "concierge medicine" or "direct primary care."[23]

Such efforts remain at the margins, however, and have little to do with the majority of health care visits. Yet, as health care utilization payment becomes increasingly complex, and efficiency as part of efforts to build health systems that are both more expansive and more efficient becomes urgent, coding follows suit, constituting a power/knowledge system to which physicians and their staffs must conform.[24] Internet message boards commonly include questions about how to get such letters, what they must say, and what the correct or more reliable nomenclature must be. There are also a myriad of examples—form letters, in essence—that physicians, physicians' office managers, and patients can use to more predictably ensure that health insurers will pay for the desired treatments. As just one example, Botox's manufacturer, Allergan, established a web platform and resource site to aid stakeholders in establishing Botox's medical necessity. Among other resources, the website provides physicians with a form letter of medical necessity. Particularly striking about the Botox letter is the balancing of the prefabricated and the customized. In a way, of course, the fact that Allergan would provide a form letter to physicians makes financial sense. But there is something odd about the formalization of this process not by way of a form, but in a letter ascribed to a particular physician. The letter illustrates the extent to which navigating the medical necessity archive requires a delicate balance of the oppositional techniques of regularity and randomization:

> I have prescribed BOTOX® neurotoxin because *provide explanation*. This treatment was medically necessary because *insert medical rationale*. The BOTOX® dosage required for the injection site in a patient of this weight is *insert appropriate dosage*.
>
> *Insert the following if appropriate:* Because there were no other patients awaiting treatment with BOTOX® neurotoxin at that time, there was an unavoidable wastage of BOTOX® totaling *indicate exact amount as number of Units*.
>
> This patient's response to the initial dose of BOTOX® has been *indicate the status, if applicable*. Based on this outcome, I plan to treat *insert patient's name* with BOTOX® *indicate the planned course of treatment and duration*. My clinical expectations for treatment with BOTOX® neurotoxin are *indicate expectations*. Follow-up is expected to involve *include expected additional evaluations and treatments*.
>
> The use of BOTOX® in this manner is well documented in literature. Copies of published clinical studies, product information, and a copy of the package insert for BOTOX® neurotoxin are enclosed for your review.[25]

Ultimately, given the instability of medical necessity discourses themselves, as well as the lack of an epistemic center within those discourses, navigating the medical necessity archive may require sheer tenacity, close attention to detail, but also attention to persuasion of the various constituencies to which the archive is designed to appeal. While physician record keeping is essential, patients may also have to become learned archivists in their own right. Blogs and other internet testimonials provide an important snapshot of patient experience.[26] A survey of these sites provides a picture of the widespread dissemination of firsthand knowledge—and the attendant production of an archive of folk wisdom—intended to help others navigate various dimensions of the American health care system.

This, in turn, requires that physicians develop complex bureaucratic mechanisms, each of which is a function of the increased complexity and contestation of medical necessity decision making itself. As these developments run their course, moreover, the medical necessity archive grows. As each such development promises efficiency and clinical effectiveness, concern intensifies over what will happen to medical necessity within shared decision-making environments.[27]

The Medical Coding Industry

A key reason for the rise of medical coding was its move from a means of tracking disease and death to regulating reimbursement schedules. In the wake of these developments, "coders were elevated out of the dark basements into the financial limelight."[28] They came to constitute a critical line of defense in payment systems. They became the unacknowledged backbone of the movement from volume care to value, since only reliable and systematic coding could track and demonstrate value.

This shift mirrors the history of medical necessity itself, in which a fairly straightforward practice of record keeping became the foundation for a system of management, transitioning from a merely descriptive role to that of a facilitative and even disciplinary regime that could be said to have reconstituted medical care delivery. The watchwords of this regime are compliance (which requires avoiding errors) and fraud (which suggests mal-intent).[29] Given the financial stakes, an industry of for-profit schools training students to reign in medical necessity decision making has arisen to master the language games through which these systems operate. This day-to-day workforce development has been accompanied by opportunities for consultants and new products promising to aid technicians in their work. Of course, given the explosion of economic and career opportunities made possible by health care reform, with employment numbers in states across the nation tied to investments in and expansion of access to health care, the timing is auspicious for the rise of such an industry. For example, Allied Schools tells potential students,

> As vital members of a medical team, medical billing professionals acquire a diverse set of skills and knowledge of medical terminology and anatomy, as well as proficiency in medical coding and billing software.

These opportunities, they note, provide employees with flexibility especially for stay-at-home parents, and have arisen out of the continual growth and complexity of medical interventions, compounded by an aging American population. The ongoing "job explosion" in medical coding is fueled as well by the need for insurance companies to continually update their claims processing procedures.[30] Aalseth adds to the excitement:

If you enjoy solving puzzles or reading mysteries, coding is just the thing. Every doctor has different methods of documenting care. New vocabulary appears in response to changing technology. Codes change annually and the rules change periodically as well. Coding is never the "same old same old."[31]

A multitude of physicians' "different methods," medical necessity's constantly-evolving discourses, and changing rules converge to create a need for an influx of coding experts. These features of medical necessity decision making and analysis are also—in Aalseth's pitch—what makes medical necessity both challenging and exciting. The anxieties associated with the release of the ICD-10, which have continued with the arrival in 2018 of the ICD-11, have come to rival the industry opportunities created by the need for mastering of the new codes. With great anxiety, of course, come opportunities for investment, service, and provision; the Web is filled with services and products promising to ease the transition across coding platforms. Indeed, it is not surprising that opportunities for profiting from the existence of these epistemic regimes should arise. In many ways, they are perfectly designed for such opportunities.

Medical Coding as Language Game

These are the preconditions and structural features of the archive. But they do not tell the whole story. Rather, a critical reading of medical coding takes note of the extent to which these processes give rise to the objects of medicine themselves, and are therefore constitutive of a broad swath of medical knowledge. As sociologists Marc Berg and Geoffrey Bowker note, the medical record "does not simply represent this body's history and geography: it is a central element in the material re-writing of these."[32] This was one of Foucault's important contributions: he noted that the observation, measurement, and recording of the clinic gave rise to new ways of knowing the medical subject, whose epistemic context was provided through the legitimation of diseases, conditions, risks, and beyond.[33]

There have been several notable moments in the politics of American health care when this trend of archival proliferation has been particularly pronounced, especially the 1991 expansion of CPT E&M guidelines for Medicare, which expanded from four to forty-four pages. These guidelines illustrate the elusive nature of the medical necessity archive. Aalseth notes:

> Put bluntly, physicians do not like these codes. They are extremely complex and difficult to interpret. In studies where physicians and coding analysts assigned E&M codes to hypothetical cases, the coding analysts agreed with expert opinion only 57% of the time, while the agreement by physicians was only 52%. This indicates a lot of gray areas in coding these services.[34]

Not only must the coding be consistent, but examinations must be undertaken in accordance with guidelines. For example, Medicare's 1995 guidelines identified four types of exams—problem-focused, expanded problem-focused, detailed, and comprehensive. Yet while physicians are expected to utilize the correct exam level, the system design assumes that the "extent of the examination performed and documented,"—which may range from a single body area to multisystem analysis,—"depends on the clinical judgment of the examiner and on the nature of the presenting problems."[35] Medical coding must persuasively capture services rendered while attending to the legitimacy of the clinical judgment of the physician rendering them. Kelly-Farwell and Favreau note, "Problems discovered during an audit are usually a result of the provider's overcoding or undercoding."[36] Persuasive medical coding, however, requires attending to both possibilities. Similarly, audits may question not only the type of procedure itself, but the place in which that procedure was carried out.[37] In other words, the reason for an exam or treatment is not enough to meet current medical necessity standards, but the place—hospitalization, office, home visit, nursing home—must be factored in as well.

Audits of medical necessity claims do tend to emphasize location. A 2011 American Hospital Association study of Medicare and Medicaid found that inadequate medical necessity determinations were by far the greatest reason (84%) for denying claims for patients' hospital care.[38] Yet, this number is also not as straightforward as it may seem, as most medical necessity denials were made based on incorrect location, not because the care itself was deemed medically unnecessary. This suggests that medical necessity is not the question, exactly, even as denials issued in response to mistakes are made in its name. Denials on the basis of medical necessity occur not only with regard to the necessity of what is done, but *where* something is done, such as an inpatient hospital setting as opposed to outpatient ambulatory settings.

It is not only the case that medical necessity determinations are highly contextualized. More than that, each layer of context opens a new epistemic front. The previous example makes it clear that ICD-10 and CPT codes thus arrive at the intersections of time and space. Aalseth counsels, "CPT codes for adult critical care are time-based: for the first 30 minutes (or less), and then for each additional 30 minutes. The physician must clearly document their time spent."[39] Medicare's Local Medical Review Policies, which are location sensitive, add variety into such decision making from a national perspective. The result is an increasing prevalence of the kind of disciplinary developments with which Foucault was concerned, where knowledge—all that we know about a certain series of medical interventions—is located within and even constituted through fields of power.[40]

As medical coding textbooks make clear, inaccurate coding can make or break a practice that is dependent upon third-party payments, as most are. Inaccurate coding also has significant consequences for patients who are either denied care or who have to pay out of pocket, if they can, to access care deemed medically unnecessary. Medical coding's promise is its ability to ensure that the argument for medical necessity is carefully and intentionally constructed. Yet this deceptively simple goal folds back on itself in surprising ways. The elusive notion of accuracy sets the stage for rhetorical slippage as well as overtly political conflict. Indeed, accuracy becomes a quite different question—specifically, a question of persuasion.

This suggests a need for rethinking how we know "the medical" as well as the necessary. To defer such questions to the authority of the archive is to commit tautology and merely empower an epistemic regime by serving as passive vehicles of power. Those who learn to navigate and manipulate the archive are all too aware that certain coding practices are likely to yield rejections. They must also understand the complexities of the medical when one considers certain challenges, such as those posed by iatrogenic interactions, coordination between providers, layers of sometimes contradictory judgments, and other dynamics that complicate coding schemas.

In mastering these dynamics, coders learn how to use coding to minimize red flags and increase the chance of "passing."[41] That some approaches are more likely to pass than others should serve as a reminder that coding is an art of persuasion. Passing is concerned with fitting in and, in a sense, creating conditions under which others may not even notice that one is there. Effective medical necessity coding seeks to accomplish a similar goal.

Consider the following narrative, from *ASC Review*, which advises hospital and health system leaders, owners and operators of ambulatory surgery centers, and leaders of orthopedic and spine practices on a range of business questions: "Spine surgeons are finding more denials based on medical necessity than in the past; insurance companies claim a procedure isn't a medical necessity because the patient doesn't fit into their criteria for coverage." And since it is challenging to persuade insurance companies that medical necessity determinations are best understood as individual assessments, surgeons must evoke case studies and outcomes data.[42] ASC advises physicians to learn to navigate insurance company guidelines and "develop a relationship with the medical director, as well as other executives, at those companies to broaden coverage in unique cases." The article also goes on to emphasize the importance of patient involvement in appeals processes. They argue, for example, that "insurance companies respond more rapidly to patients being upset about their care than the physicians," and counsel physicians to "be available to do the peer-to-peer reviews and don't take 'no' for an answer."

Importantly, ASC emphasizes the importance of relationship building. Conceptually, this places such actors within the rhetorical domain of ethos, where persuasive appeals are dependent upon the credibility of speakers, instead of logos, where rational argumentation is emphasized. Once credibility is established, particular arguments may be made. "The key going forward," they argue, "will be to overcome the hammer spine surgery is facing with the perception of over-utilization." Note that the concern here is with perception. Over-utilization, in this view, is not always a fact, but certain procedures and certain areas of medicine may be more or less subject to misperceptions, and must therefore attend to them. This casts medical necessity in a light not unlike that of tax services that indicate and seek to minimize the likelihood of an audit. The risks one takes in coding in a certain way, especially where reimbursement is at stake, is directly related to the liability one may face in the process. Aggressive and conservative coding strategies each come with distinct risks and rewards.

Another example is illustrated by an online article published by the American College of Osteopathic Family Physicians to help osteopathic practitioners successfully code for osteopathic manipulative treatment (OMT), a historically-marginalized series of treatments that are particular to the world of osteopathic care. Entitled "OMT Coding Strategies to Boost Your Bottom Line," the article explains the importance of distinguishing evaluation and management from treatments, but also issues a caveat regarding language:

> In terms of treatment options, it is imperative that we are consistent in our terminology. Semantics matter and as physicians we provide treatment not therapy. A few years ago a prominent payor took a stance nationally to deny payment for craniosacral therapy. This was likely done, in large part, to halt therapists' reimbursement for craniosacral therapy. However OCF or osteopathy in the cranial field is not therapy, but treatment and is still readily reimbursed.[43]

While these resources are directed at health practitioners, others directly address patients. Medical advice websites are chock full of message boards in which patients attempt to figure out what is and is not medically necessary under their particular plans, and where a denial has been issued, strategizing ways to sneak a procedure or prescription in under the radar. Such online forums underscore the multiple audiences within medical necessity's persuasive dimensions.

Particularly striking about these forums is their often open, even brazen admission that convincing powers-that-be of the medical necessity of certain forms of care is closer to a game than being a principled matter of some procedures being empirically medically necessary and others not. Indeed, the challenges of medical coding have given rise to a large body of internet information intended to help—(though coach might be a more accurate word)—coders ensure payment. In the field of dermatology, Inga Ellzey notes, "The sole use of [an ICD code for inflamed seborrheic kerotosis, a benign skin wart] is insufficient to justify lesion removal without medical record documentation of the patient's symptoms and physical findings." Accordingly, the "medical record must show that the lesion(s) was symptomatic in order for the treatment to be charged to an insurance company." Ellzey offers advice for justifying dermatological treatments, noting subtle differences in terminology that determine whether or not procedures will be considered medically necessary. She counsels: "Use the term 'shave removal,' not 'shave excision' or 'shave biopsy,'" since these terminologies depart from coding requirements, even if the terms are functionally synonymous.[44] Yet, while the terminological advice is issued under the guise of accuracy, the difference is linked to the terms' relative persuasiveness in support of medical necessity, even when they mark the same procedure. Such moments run the risk of detaching themselves entirely from worldly referents to serve a broader rhetorical function.[45] In other words, the strategy that coding experts counsel amounts to one of mastering the language games required to gain persuasive leverage within contemporary medical necessity debates.

Such mastery requires commanding a lexicon beyond the discourse of medical necessity. It also requires keeping not only cosmetic, experimental, social, and elective care at bay, but considerations such as distinguishing medically necessary or "therapeutic" abortions from the more politically-charged rhetoric of "abortion on demand."[46] The epistemic determination of medical necessity arises out of the archive insofar as it is distinguished from various "others," which are not merely excluded from medical necessity but serve as what critical theorists call its "constitutive outside," or what it is not. Distinction from this "other" is critical for securing treatments for patients. The discourse of medical necessity, in other words, is concerned first and foremost with navigating a field of power that leaves the delivery of care hanging in the balance.

The Rhetoric of Accuracy: Medical Coding as Persuasion

I have suggested that defining our way out of medical necessity's language games is often a fool's errand. It is nonetheless the case that definitional debates about correct coding stand at the center of the question of what actually happened during a given clinical event. I have also established that such questions of language are always both constrained by and made legible through systems of power/knowledge that contain a wide range of medical phenomena. These include financial considerations, malpractice, religious and other cultural concerns, and the broader politics of evidence-based medicine. The phenomenological question of what a clinician "did" is not simple.

For example, John Lantos recounts the quite different ways in which an event may be cast. The following considerations were raised in a case in which he provided expert testimony:

> It was a difficult labor, with a double-footling breech presentation. When the mother had arrived at the hospital two tiny, bluish feet were protruding from her vagina. (Here we have to be careful with our language. She's not a 'mother' until her baby is born. Should we call her a 'pregnant woman'? a 'woman in labor'? a 'patient'? a 'pregnant health care consumer'?) The choice of words colors the case; no word is morally neutral. Each swirls the current, nudges the raft.[47]

Such cases do not only raise questions about what is and isn't medically necessary; they also raise questions about what a physician did or did not do at the most microtechnical of levels. Lantos notes that physicians working in especially high-pressure situations—in his case, a neonatal intensive care unit—operate in environments marked by complex spacio-temporal conditions, namely tiny babies embedded in fast-changing and sometimes elusive conditions.[48] By design, these conditions require snap judgments made in fields of contingency. The mode of judgment is probabilistic rather than syllogistic, in a way that belies necessity's rhetorical promise. Lantos juxtaposes those conditions with the black and white standard many lawyers demand when presenting cases in front of juries for medical malpractice cases. The result is that two quite different perspectives get put under the same rhetorical umbrella of whether or not what was necessary was done, including whether it was necessary, appropriate, contingent, and so forth. Each of these terms, as I have discussed, is itself problematic and in need of definition.

Strategies for effective coding are therefore not—as one might assume—merely concerned with accuracy. Instead, they seek to control, tame, and contain an order of discourse. In so doing, coders must tarry with extant systems of power/knowledge. Given the epistemic nature of medicine, which concerns human beings rather than logic, precision is often a moving target, a function of an imperfect process. To reflect this imperfection, medical coding must be understood to address a process that seeks not to promulgate truths, but to cultivate legitimacy—with each case contributing to the possible legitimization or de-legitimization of particular codes. Necessity is the outcome of a complex of discourses that are infused with value. As is the case with any complex coding schema, error can enter into the process at any point. But error is understood, in this view, in a quite different way, as a simple failure to correspond to truth. Rhetorical analysis helps us to see the degree to which error is a function of a failure to persuade. It does not get us closer to understanding the truth of necessity, but rather helps us to notice the rhetorical production of truth itself. This is consistent with Derridean analysis which, as Stanley Fish has noted, "does not uncover the operations of rhetoric in order to reach the Truth; rather, it continually uncovers the truth of rhetorical operations, the truth that all operations, including the operation of deconstruction itself, are rhetorical."[49]

The medical coding industry, with its deep bench of experts, schools, and technologies, promises to produce a regularity and predictability that, in turn, can yield persuasive effects. Sometimes this goal is made explicit. Inga Ellzey advises, for example, "You must be judicious about your documentation patterns. Not every patient can have the exact same symptoms. That will send up a red flag." Hence, "every lesion you treat cannot be irritated. That will certainly not fly in a carrier audit."[50]

It is, of course, not only the case that coding is situated within broader considerations of power within health care systems. More specifically, learning to correctly situate codes is a critical skill on which patients' access to care may hinge, and practices' fiscal stability may rise and fall. At stake is not only the financial status of practices, but their credibility. Berg and Bowker note, for example:

> The record not only plays a generative role in the organization of the clinic, it also legitimates this organization's design. As we have pointed out above, the record tells the story of the *work* this body politic performs. One way of evaluating the record has been to see every record as a description of a structure of a working organization operating at peak efficiency. Thus, record keepers are advised that the purpose of the record is to tell a story that begins with admission, describes [a] diagnostic process, goes on to treatment, and ends with discharge, or (even more "complete" from the medical record keepers' perspective) death. In this case the outcome of the record is again the meta-affirmation that allopathic medicine works—and, ipso facto, that the sites where medicine is performed

work. Every record, as individual as may be, is through its very form, testament to this assertion of success.[51]

But what does "accuracy" mean in this context? That accuracy in medical necessity decision making operates as a mode of persuasion is clear enough. But the issue can be read in two quite different ways. A first reading suggests a need for attending to differences between patients and making often subtle distinctions between disparate conditions, largely in response to what Ellzey, for example, views as a tendency for dermatologists to copy and paste patient information from record to record—a practice known as "cloning"—which creates an appearance of consistency across patient profiles.[52] It is this consistency, and not a lack of consistency, that produces the "red flag." A second reading, however, suggests that distinctions must be made, not because they are clinically justified, but because a track record of claims requires a delicate balance of predictability and particularity. A paradox stands at the center of what we might call the coding and necessity "justification movement," which aims at systemization in the name of accuracy and guarding against fraud, but balks when things get *too* systematic or regular—a paradoxical kind of system that must appear systematic, but not overly standardized. Either way, one cannot ascertain whether determinations are made in the name of more specific clinical judgments, or to produce the appearance of specificity where none is required. Another way to understand this, in the language of rhetoric, is that utilization review must be persuaded of claims' legitimacy, but coders must not appear too persuasive or too eager to convince.

This suggests the need for a series of corollary strategies to amend the advice to "Always code to the highest level of specificity."[53] The result is that medical necessity determinations that escape the perception of fraud must adhere to certain rhetorical patterns—orderly in some senses, particularly in relation to ICD coding and the use of certain preferred terminologies, but disorderly in others so as not to appear to be an outcome of physicians using medical necessity determinations for purposes that providers consider illegitimate. In other words, successful medical coding obscures the existence of the language game of medical coding itself. It is only as a last resort—and at considerable risk of disrupting this appearance—that a coder should turn to catch-all codes such as Not Otherwise Specified and Not Elsewhere Classified.[54] Aalseth explains, "Sometimes there is no existing CPT code that adequately describes the procedure performed . . . due to new techniques, additional technological developments, or procedures performed on anomalous anatomy caused by congenital malformations."[55] CPT includes an "unlisted" code ending in "99" to denote an exception which, of course, may be rejected for payment. Ellzey predicts that the growth of electronic records will excite auditors' scrutiny of medical necessity determinations, in part because such systems lend themselves to easier analysis. But the thrust of her argument is to suggest that with some careful attention to the codes, as well as specific trends in the language of medical necessity, audits will be easy. Here, again, I wish to highlight the detachment of medical necessity coding from more grounded medical debates, and the emphasis on gaming, where the point of medical coding is not accuracy in any empirical sense, but winning. Particularly striking is medical coding textbooks' lack of attention to the filtering process that underpins (and even gives rise to) the codes themselves. Within the context of professional training, the discourse of medical necessity is treated largely uncritically, as a purely functional discourse that is not always implicated in shaping medical knowledge itself.

Judgment and Coding

The difficulty that clinicians and their support staff have in navigating these complexities underscores the complicated nature of medical necessity decision making as well as the unique competencies that documenting medical necessity requires. It also sheds light on the unstable nature of the archive from which medical necessity arises, regardless of particular coding practices. Specifically, there is a tendency to tack back and forth between the pursuit of stable medical necessity standards and the inherent unpredictability of medical necessity, especially as interpreted by health care providers and other stakeholders. Peter Jensen, a nephrologist and author of articles on medical necessity, advises, "When it comes to selecting the appropriate level of care for any encounter, medical necessity trumps everything else, including the documentation of history, physical exam and medical decision-making."[56] Not even so-called bulletproof documentation in diagnosis and treatment will carry weight in the absence of proving medical necessity. Jensen recommends the following shorthand: "If you feel silly asking a question during the history or performing elements of a physical exam, it probably means you have wandered off the path of medical necessity."[57] This echoes other views that consider medical necessity "more of a euphemism for physician habit than a scientific yardstick."[58] Bluntly put: why would silliness be a reliable epistemic indicator at all?

Things are more complicated and less certain when strategies concern not only avoiding care that may be deemed medically unnecessary,—but *proving* medical necessity's presence in positive terms. Jensen notes that ICD codes are "the first line of defense when it comes to medical necessity," and advises using all four code spaces provided by standard Medicare billing to provide the code with additional epistemic support. He calls the first code the "power code" because it signifies an overarching diagnosis, which is then supported with subsequent codes to specify treatment protocols. The promise is that careful coding will adequately translate physicians' orders into the proper bureaucratic language to ensure payment: "Let medical necessity guide the care you provide, document that care accurately and code based on your documentation. This will help ensure fewer claims denials and appropriate care for your patients."[59]

But what is the nature of the relationship between the supposedly objective medical necessity of an encounter and the coding regime that requires specific coding and documentation regimes to pass muster? Echoing Foucault's "clinical gaze," which immediately "*perceives a spectacle*,"[60] Jensen lets "medical decision-making point [him] toward what [he thinks] will be the appropriate code." Ultimately, however, he makes an empirical claim as the codes themselves, and not physicians' judgments, determine medical necessity. The physician cannot guarantee that even the most scrupulous coding regime will yield a persuasive medical necessity determination. This leads Jensen to concede the limits of controlling medical necessity's discursive boundaries. What, he asks, is the difference between "necessary" treatments and a "service" that a physician "feels" is "important"?[61] One health consultant offers some practical advice: "Don't code from perception; code from fact, from what's written down," adding that some optometrists apply cookbook coding, incorrectly using the same codes for patients with similar diagnoses. "A lot of optometrists get their coding knowledge from colleagues and going to seminars, then apply things improperly in many cases."[62]

Those who advocate taking medical coding more seriously tend to fall into a pattern, namely that they are in the business of developing and selling new technologies for making medical coding both more efficient and more accurate. Such advocates often argue against relying on intuition, appearances, or judgment. Their companies stand to gain from the development of new technologies for medical coding, but must be careful in depending upon them. Yet, consistently, on internet blogs and industry web pages, the rhetorical claim persists that coding is about compliance, not profits. Skillful coding, in other words, is billed as consistent with the delivery of quality patient care. The claim is that there is no money to be made in bad (or bad faith) coding. Truth is compatible with financial bottom lines.

Upon further inspection, however, this does not always appear to be the case. Controversies over the use of intensity-modulated radiation therapy (IMRT), a targeted but expensive technology for treating breast cancer, illustrates a structural problem at work. A study conducted by the National Cancer Institute found that during a five-year period, IMRT drove up the cost of radiation treatment by more than double. This cost might be understandable but for the fact that, "tumor characteristics were not strongly associated with an increased use of IMRT, suggesting that it was not being adopted to address a perceived medical concern." As a result, the researchers conclude that widespread use of IMRT "would appear to confirm the suspicion of many, both within and outside of the healthcare industry, that medical decision-making is too heavily influenced by reimbursement rather than medical necessity."[63]

As I have noted, prominent authors such as David Goldhill attribute a constantly expanding conception of medical necessity to our dependence on third-party "surrogates" with "perverse" incentives, especially companies with financial stakes in such an expansive conception.[64] The result is that rising health care costs and expanded need have made third-party consultation and oversight central to medical necessity debates. The promise of these consultations seems to be—as they advertise—that their expertise can tame unwieldy medical necessity discourses and secure health provider revenue streams. Trade publications spotlight companies specializing in the scrutiny of medical necessity claims. A press release from the claims review division of Cypress Benefit Administrators explains, for example, "While many [accounting] discrepancies relate to being billed the wrong rate or too much for a single service, others are associated with more complex issues like medical necessity." Through an increasingly common phenomenon known as "retrospective peer independent review," they report finding evidence of unnecessary treatments ordered and considerable financial waste. According to the CEO, "It's not just instances of obvious overpricing that we watch for on behalf of our employer clients. Our claim specialists are trained to review charges from a medical necessity perspective and flag anything that seems excessive or out of the ordinary." As such efforts become increasingly common, "The days of ordering extra, unneeded tests to help supplement the cost of expensive equipment or avoid potential malpractice suits are coming to an end."[65] At the same time, the existence of these kind of organizations make clear that the epistemic questions raised by medical necessity give rise not only to a system for organizing medical knowledge, but an industry.

Coding Unnecessary Care

As I argued, medical necessity's persuasiveness depends upon its reception by others, as well as their willingness to legitimize its definitional boundaries. Perhaps this is why though electronic medical records and other digital systems can be useful, practitioners should not put too much faith in their ability to mediate or settle the politics of medical necessity. This is not only the case because "computer systems will never be able to mimic the judgment and insight necessary to accurately assess medical necessity," but because the users of such systems still must navigate a series of constraints to establish medical necessity. The limitations of computers generally, and electronic medical records in particular, in taming the excitable nature of medical necessity decision making suggest that technology is the promise of, as well as a central paradox within, the broader politics of medical necessity. On some level, like language itself,[66] even the most complex algorithms fail to account for the diversity and richness of medical questions.

Yet, as with most phenomena read through a Foucauldian lens, technology is double-edged. As new technologies raise questions (as well as expectations) about medicine's potential to address health problems, they systematize medical phenomena by creating a new epistemic order. At the center of this order is the carving out of a distinction between the medical and the nonmedical—that is, medicalization. But, as we know, these are not mere technical distinctions, but carry with them the introduction of a value-laden epistemic order that, through technical, scientific, and other means, obscures its own value-laden basis. Derrida noted this phenomenon with regard to email, but the point applies to other technological developments as well:

It is not only a technique, in the ordinary and limited sense of the term: at an unprecedented rhythm, in quasi-instantaneous fashion, this instrumental possibility of production, of printing, of conservation, and of destruction of the archive must inevitably be accompanied by juridical and thus political transformations. These affect nothing less than property rights, publishing and reproduction rights.[67]

Derrida conjures not only the immediate impact that technology is having on the archive—which extends logically to the medical archive as well—but ethical questions such as privacy and the ownership of one's records that are always bound up in technological developments. As Derrida puts it, "what is no longer archived in the same way is no longer lived in the same way."[68] The archive changes the nature of things themselves. In Foucauldian terms, the archive creates subjects through its discursive processing.

As we would expect, with this power come tools for opportunity. The result is a fast-developing and ever-expanding industry of new products promising to tame and navigate these new forms of life. For example, 3M Health Information Systems, the manufacturer of medical necessity validation software for coders, notes the following:

> Uncompensated medically unnecessary services total billions of dollars per year. Without accurate medical necessity checking, you could find your reimbursement entangled in claim denials and delays. Plus, accurate validation can help you determine when to issue an ABN form, letter of medical necessity or other noncoverage documentation appropriately so you can comply with medical necessity guidelines.[69]

The software promises to help users to code interventions so that they pass muster vis-à-vis medical necessity. It does this by offering a series of tools for editing codes and ensuring that they are drawing upon the most up-to-date developments, such as changes in local medical review policies. Presumably, like tax software aiming to prevent an audit, such software must stay up to date on the latest regulatory practices as well. Taken as a whole, such technologies are staked in the promise of making medical necessity more predictable and outcomes less unpredictable. To be successful, they must be continually updated and track shifting forces in the world of medical decision making that they attempt to navigate.

Several conclusions stem from these observations. On the one hand, weak documentation could signify insufficient attention to detail in the deliberation over and delivery of care. Whatever the cause, from fraud to mere poor documentation, problems with documentation open doors to a number of practical and political questions. On the other hand, health providers who regularly pay out large sums of money for services have reason to be concerned about the use of unnecessary care, not only because such care could be construed as a luxury instead of a necessity, but because unnecessary care can weaken health outcomes in addition to raising costs. This focus on coding *for* medical necessity makes clear that there is often a wide gap between the service or equipment provided—which may or may not be considered medically necessary—and documentation. The persuasive abilities of the techniques I have described are concerned with obscuring this gap.

Consider, for example, the following question: while wheelchair technology has developed far beyond the hand-propelled chairs that patients have used for decades, are electric wheelchairs medically necessary? Motivated by a finding that between 1999 and 2003, Medicare payments for electric wheelchairs increased from $259 million to $1.2 billion annually, or about 350 percent, the HHS's Office of Inspector General found that, "61 percent of power wheelchairs provided to Medicare beneficiaries in the first half of 2007 were medically unnecessary or had claims that lacked sufficient documentation to determine medical necessity."[70] The report provides two separate lines of reasoning. The first is that in 9 percent of cases, the reasons provided by physicians were deemed incorrect, where CMS found that medical necessity claims were incorrectly established. 2 percent of these cases were found to require less expensive equipment, such as manual wheelchairs, while 7 percent were found to warrant a different type of power wheelchair. The second line of reasoning notes that 52 percent of claims were "insufficiently documented to determine whether the power wheelchairs were medically necessary,"[71] which points to an epistemological as well as bureaucratic thicket in which one cannot distinguish the necessary from the unnecessary, not because such determinations are impossible to make, but because they require near-flawless and extensive documentation that often falls by the wayside as it is operationalized in actual health care contexts. In other words, the most common medical necessity denials are not sensational cases of fraud or neglect, such as intentionally-administered unnecessary surgery or illegal prescription practices,[72] but the result of incorrect documentation. More often than not, questions about medical necessity exist only in the negative, as something undocumented and not proven rather than exposed as unnecessary.[73]

A series of recent controversies about cardiac procedures illustrate these dynamics. In 2012, for example, a whistle-blowing nurse reported to the ethics officer of a Florida hospital that unnecessary heart catheterizations and stents were being utilized by hospital staff. A follow-up report confirmed the nurse's allegations, which linked the findings to the hospital's parent organization, the Hospital Corporation of America (HCA), which owned 163 facilities at the time. The report found that "the nurse's complaint was far from the only evidence that unnecessary—even dangerous—procedures were taking place at some HCA hospitals, driving up costs and increasing profits." Interestingly, the report did not unearth evidence that unnecessary care had been delivered, but rather an absence of proof in that some of HCA's physicians "were unable to justify many of the procedures they were performing [and] in some cases . . . made misleading statements in medical records that made it appear the procedures were necessary."[74] About half of the cardiac catheterizations at one hospital were found to have been performed on patients without significant heart disease. HCA's response to the report sheds light on the politics of the situation:

> The cardiologists say the reviews of their work did not accurately reflect the care they provided, and HCA says the reviews "are not, by any means, definitive." . . . HCA says it took whatever steps were necessary to improve patient care. It also said "significant actions were taken to investigate areas of concern, to bring in independent reviewers, and to take action where necessary."
>
> Details about the procedures and the company's knowledge of them are contained in thousands of pages of confidential memos, e-mail correspondence among executives, transcripts from hearings and reports from outside consultants examined by *The Times*, as well as interviews with doctors and others. A review of those communications reveals that rather than asking whether patients had been harmed or whether regulators needed to be contacted,

hospital officials asked for information on how the physicians' activities affected the hospitals' bottom line.[75]

The very idea that there could be a "definitive" reading of the report is tenuous at best. Notice also the group's promise to "take action where necessary," a promise to attend to professional imperatives in the interest of ensuring medical necessity. In other words, if medical necessity is approached without care, the integrity of larger professional systems is at risk.

A final example comes from an HHS review of hemodialysis services billed to Medicare. According to the review, though one hundred services reviewed met Medicare requirements for medical necessity, eleven did not adequately document that a physician was present during hemodialysis, as required by Medicare rules. Sixty-one did not adequately document the medical necessity for repeated evaluation of patients by physicians, as Medicare requires.[76] All told, the study determined that $151,566 out of the $542,996 total paid out for those one hundred cases should have been rejected, not because the procedures weren't medically necessary, but because they were poorly or inadequately documented.

At a time when American health care politics is increasingly focused on expanded access, improved outcomes, and cost containment, health care experts are beginning to get a handle on the big picture of unnecessary health care services—even as the unnecessary continues to elude. In 2018, for example, the Washington Health Alliance released a comprehensive report about unnecessary health care services entitled "First, Do No Harm." After an examination of forty-seven "common treatment approaches known by the medical community to be overused," the report found that more than 45 percent of the services examined were of "low value," meaning "likely wasteful or wasteful," with those services delivered to approximately 1.3 million individuals.[77] From these findings, the report's authors issued a five-part call to action that recommended that Washington State actively engage in a discussion about overuse in assessing the value of health care services, calling on "clinical leaders" to lead efforts to reduce overuse, and stating that the concepts of "choosing wisely" and a commitment to shared decision making should be made the foundation of provider–patient communications. As one mechanism to encourage these developments, the report reasserts the importance of paying increasingly for value instead of volume, which requires that provider contracts include measures of overuse—"and not just measures of access and underuse"—as they support a movement toward evidence-based care.[78] Such reports are likely to become increasingly common within the current and coming health policy dynamic. The question is whether findings that much or even most health care spending is unnecessary will provoke a critical, pointed, and open debate about the meaning of medical necessity.

Work in the medical necessity archive is a slog. For structural reasons, the techniques on offer to navigate it do not guarantee success. My focus on the archive and the coding process that creates it suggests that actors cannot be secondarily concerned with the rhetorical dimensions of medical care, or an analysis of the power relations that shape it, but must attend to them directly. As the current organization of health care requires attention to systems in which physicians are an important part—but nevertheless only a part—medical coding must be considered a distinct voice and not simply a source of pressure on physicians' voices. We must attend, instead, to the values that end up being deposited in the archive, to notice how they are written, contested, altered, and enforced. The philosopher Norman Daniels recounts the following in a dated but useful example:

> In the Clinton administration's effort in 1993 to introduce universal insurance coverage, I served on the Ethics Working Group. At one point, David Eddy and I were asked to develop a definition of "medical necessity." Our definition omitted nontherapeutic abortion from the category of "medically necessary treatments of disease or dysfunction" since a normal pregnancy was not pathological in any way. Some task force members insisted that we redefine the concept of medical necessity to include (nontherapeutic) abortions automatically. When we asked how that could be done without also counting as medically necessary cosmetic surgery for noses deemed unattractive, we were told that the cases were different. On discussion, the differences had nothing to do with normal or abnormal functioning, but rather with other reasons for considering one intervention more important than the other. No one suggested that something became a disease by being an unwanted condition.[79]

As these layers of complexity accumulate, the philosophically and legally vexing question of proving (and documenting) intention becomes increasingly important. As we have seen, the nature of the medical necessity archive makes it difficult to differentiate insidious intent from error. News reports are filled with instances of so-called medical necessity fraud.[80] Within the politics of medical necessity, however, fraud is an interpretive complexity rather than cause for simple blame. Indeed, the manner in which intent is ascribed depends in large part on which rhetorical register—legal, moral, philosophical, biomedical, community-oriented, economic, and social—one operates. Just as problematically, one usually moves simultaneously in more than one at any given time.

More important than any one assessment is a general disposition that always encounters and approaches the archive,—as well as the processes through which it is constituted,—as a process composed of rhetorical moves within a field of interpretation and power. This chapter seeks to explain, above all, why there is no purely linguistic or definitional, predictive, or technological way to solve the problem of defining medical necessity. Far from solving the problem of medical necessity, medical coding, central as it is to health care documentation and financing, creates a whole series of questions about medical epistemology, the nature of medicine, and the aims of health care. The industry that has arisen to strategize and clarify the aims of coding, and to make the process more predictable, will continue to do its work. But it does not solve the problem of medical necessity precisely because it treats the concept as a purely technical matter. In so doing, the medical coding industry misses what is most interesting about medical necessity itself, namely the intertwined nature of facts and values in policy debates.[81]

3

"No Legitimate Use"

Marijuana and the Bounds of the Medical

The politics of medical necessity has significant consequences far beyond access to medically-sanctioned services and goods. Beyond access, it plays an important role in shaping the very idea of "the medical" as a clinical, rhetorical, financial, gendered, and even moral and religious concern. This question of conceptual reach and multiplicity is of tremendous consequence to the legal and political boundaries through which we understand medicine. It suggests that we can fruitfully study medical necessity as a question of medical politics as well as an exercise in conceptual boundary drawing and contestation. The outcomes stemming from the politics of medical necessity bear on medical epistemology as much as they do on medical politics.

As I emphasized in previous chapters, the boundary between the legitimately and illegitimately "medical" constitutes medical necessity's central political theater. This makes sense since, as scholars have documented, the legitimacy of practices and institutions are grounded in rhetorical practices and strategies.[1] Policing these boundaries are a host of actors, from physicians and patients to lawmakers and advocates for change, as well as law enforcement officers and institutions, federal agencies, and courts. Within medical necessity's broader politics, one important thread of the story this book seeks to tell is how various actors jockey for position in medical necessity debates and how those actors shape medical necessity's ultimate meaning.

Here again the question is not one of any would-be real or true necessity, but concerns an outcome of rhetorical contests that are, depending on their persuasive effects, afforded the force of policy. The question of medical marijuana advances our understanding of the politics of medical necessity by infusing the analysis with an admixture of moralistic skepticism about marijuana itself, half-baked claims about benefits and risks, and legal considerations. In engaging marijuana's significance to these debates, and to appreciate the rhetorical layers at work in medical marijuana debates, it is again useful to let the actors speak. Consider, for example, the normative judgments sprinkled throughout comments made by Lieutenant Richard Sigley of Tulare County, California, who headed up the county's narcotics enforcement efforts. According to Sigley, "some of the plants being grown here at sites with valid and phony medical recommendations are ending up as part of the street drug trade in Utah, Illinois, Arizona and other states." Just as medical coding is characterized by a delicate balance of regularity and irregularity, law enforcement knows that the legitimacy of these documents is at issue. Sigley reports, for example, that officers "see copies of the same medical recommendations [essentially a physician letter] posted at multiple sites, and the plants can number in the hundreds or more than a thousand—well beyond the numbers listed on the recommendations." Sigley declares emphatically, "I've yet to see a legitimate marijuana grow with medical necessity. . . . And the reason I don't see those is because the ones doing it legally and for medical necessity, they aren't the ones planting 99 plants in their backyard. Because if they need it for medical necessity, they can get by with two plants annually."[2] In Sigley's telling, the rhetoric of medical necessity is possessed of moral hazard. It is a discourse to be used deceptively by those with an entirely separate agenda than that which is normally signaled by medical discourse. Worse still: medical discourse is evoked as a cover.

Paradoxically, the introduction of a particular threshold of legitimacy—the "properly" medical—creates fields of suspicion precisely where it is intended to clarify. While the theme of suspicion is common to medical necessity debates generally, in medical marijuana debates it is distinguished by its affiliation with a different category—recreation—rather than cosmetic, experimental, or other markers of unnecessary medicine. Though medical arguments about marijuana have existed for decades, a more concerted and clinically-grounded focus on the plant's medical uses is of relatively recent vintage. Historically, the most commonly encountered arguments in defense of legalization were made in the name not of therapeutic benefits but political liberty and limited government. However, after years of attempts on the part of promarijuana groups such as the National Organization for the Reform of Marijuana Laws to advocate for marijuana legalization, many groups steered their pursuit of recreational marijuana laws toward a comparatively uncontroversial focus on marijuana's potential medical benefits.

The 1990s saw an uptick of arguments in support of legalization for medical purposes. Advocates claim that marijuana's purported medical benefits are many. Many physicians, and an ever-growing list of states that have legalized medical marijuana,[3] see uses for marijuana in treating pain, nausea, vomiting associated with chemotherapy, severe weight loss associated with AIDS and AIDS treatments, and relieving intraocular pressure resulting from glaucoma.[4] As we should expect, however, marijuana's medical benefits are contested.[5] For example, a 1999 Institute of Medicine report concludes that "the benefits of smoking marijuana were limited by the toxic effects of the smoke," but still recommends "that the drug be given under close supervision to patients who do not respond to other therapies."[6] The report also rejects the premise that marijuana functioned as a "gateway" drug.

Marijuana's place within the broader culture amplifies the perception of its risks, although all remedies carry risk. In 2017, however, the National Academy of Medicine (formerly the Institute of Medicine) published a comprehensive report on the evidence regarding the health effects of cannabis, with research recommendations. Among hundreds of findings regarding the current state of cannabis research, the report's authors called for the initiation of a "national cannabis research agenda" composed of wide-ranging research, including clinical and observational research, health policy and health economics, and public health and public safety. Several of the report's recommendations concerned establishing parameters for studying cannabis, as well as strategies for addressing the current barriers, including legal barriers, to the advancement of the cannabis research agenda.[7] In short, the report can be interpreted as making the most basic claim one can make about marijuana and medical necessity, namely that we need to be able to study cannabis to make medical claims about it.

Yet, beyond the available or emerging science, medical claims concerning marijuana arise in a field of social and political contention as well, for two related reasons. First, marijuana's place in American culture makes it a topic laden with meanings that both support and undermine medical arguments. Second, and compounding the first, is the basic fact that all medical claims are contestable, especially insofar as all remedies possess risks that must be weighed against benefits. The degree to which such claims are contested in turn depends upon the level of controversy they provoke. In other words, comparatively uncontroversial treatments (the setting of a fractured bone, for example, or the insertion of a heart stent) do not evoke the kind of critical disposition that medical marijuana does. Such treatments lack the kind of excitable discourse that marijuana, abortion, and other politically-charged and contentious issues produce.

Pre-CSA, CSA, and After Effects

The regulation of marijuana was shaped by a number of important legislative developments over the last century. The most important early development was the Towns-Boylan Act of 1914, passed by the New York state legislature, which prohibited drugs believed to be habit-forming, with the exception of those acquired by prescription. In a way, the story of medical marijuana mirrors that of medical necessity itself. It first arose as a discourse tied to physicians' authority, with the prescription serving as the critical authorization mechanism. Towns-Boylan also took aim at certain classifications of physicians, prohibiting addicted physicians from practicing and noting that the "medical profession does nothing to protect the public against the irresponsible doctor," thereby creating new mechanisms for disbarment from practice.[8]

Marijuana remained largely within states' purview until 1971 when the federal Controlled Substances Act (CSA) took effect.[9] The CSA classifies marijuana as a Schedule I narcotic, which means that the federal government holds that the drug has "no currently-accepted medical use in the United States" and lacks "accepted safety for use of the substance under medical supervision."[10] As the extensive literature on the CSA and medical marijuana makes clear, the process by which marijuana was scheduled was unorthodox, with Congress foregoing input from the attorney general, as well as the biomedical and broader health sciences community.[11]

To understand post-CSA developments in the medical necessity of marijuana, it is important to consider the issues raised in key cases, since it is in the details that we can see the politics of medical necessity most clearly. It is here, as well, that dominant rhetorical patterns concerning marijuana are codified in legal discourse. Marijuana advocates tend to mark the beginning of post-CSA legal developments with *United States v. Randall* in 1971, which made its way to the U.S. Supreme Court after a federal judge ruled that Randall, who was suffering from glaucoma, could use marijuana out of medical necessity. It was the first such dispensation since 1937.[12] The judge wrote, "While blindness was shown by competent medical testimony to be the otherwise inevitable result of defendant's disease, no adverse effects from the smoking of marijuana have been demonstrated. . . . Medical evidence suggests that the medical prohibition is not well-founded." Expert testimony supported Randall's position and maintained that his right to preserve sight outweighed government interest. His defense cited two important abortion rights cases, *Roe v. Wade* and *Doe v. Bolton*, as well as *Rutherford v. United States* (which approved the use of laetrile, a now dismissed supposed alternative treatment for cancer patients[13]) as the basis of their case.

In 1978 Randall sued the Food and Drug Administration (FDA), the National Institute on Drug Abuse, the Department of Justice, and the Department of Health, Education, and Welfare because, despite the court's holding, he failed to secure access. The settlement became the basis for the FDA's Compassionate Investigational New Drug program, which allowed patients under certain conditions to acquire marijuana through a lengthy application process. This program expanded to include HIV-positive individuals, though President George H. W. Bush ended it in 1992 as part of an antidrug campaign. As of 2011, four Americans continued to receive medical marijuana through the program.[14] Some scholars maintain that the program closing in the early years of the AIDs crisis gave rise to the medical marijuana movement.[15]

Legal developments continued as political agitation began to gain traction. In 1979, in *State v. Diana*, an appellate court in the state of Washington heard a possession case. The arresting officers responded to a domestic disturbance and a woman outside told the police that her husband, inside, was "crazy" and armed. When the police entered, they saw the appellant, Samuel Diana, lying on the floor, moaning and talking. The police, who claimed that they believed that Diana was in danger, approached and discovered marijuana near where Diana was talking on the phone. Diana appealed on two accounts: unlawful entry by the police; and the refusal of the court to entertain a medical necessity defense. The appeals court believed the police entered correctly given the circumstances—so the marijuana was admissible—but upheld Diana's medical necessity defense, which he made on the basis of therapy for multiple sclerosis. The case was remanded for a reconsideration of Diana's medical necessity defense, and the court asserted that the trial court must recognize such a defense if,

(1) the defendant reasonably believed his use of marijuana was necessary to minimize the effects of multiple sclerosis; (2) the

benefits derived from its use are greater than the harm sought to be prevented by the controlled substances law; and (3) no drug is as effective in minimizing the effects of the disease.[16]

The lower courts affirmed the appellate court's finding. However, a 1998 challenge, *State of Washington v. Williams*, reversed the decision's holding that a common-law medical necessity defense existed, particularly because determinations of marijuana's medical benefits required legislative action, and the legislature had affirmed the standard set by the CSA that marijuana had no accepted medical uses.[17] Yet in the same year, Washington State legalized medical marijuana by ballot initiative, negating the force of these prior state-level questions. The back and forth of the Washington case illustrates the tensions that exist between legal-scientific judgments and political processes, the latter of which can trump the former.

Gonzales v. Raich (1996) marks the most extensive federal judicial engagement with the question of medical marijuana to date. After Raich's home was raided and his plants seized by federal agents, Raich and co-defendant Monson sought relief from the U.S. attorney general and the head of the DEA, which would have blocked enforcement of the CSA "to the extent it prevents them from possessing, obtaining, or manufacturing cannabis for their personal medical use." Raich and Monson sought relief under the argument that the CSA violated not only the doctrine of medical necessity, but the U.S. Constitution's commerce clause and the Fifth Amendment's due process clause, as well as the Ninth and Tenth Amendments. As such, *Raich* draws upon constitutional as well as long-standing arguments regarding last resorts and fundamental rights.[18] Raich and Monson both suffered from multiple and serious medical conditions that their physicians, having tried a range of remedies, determined were best treated by marijuana. As *Raich* notes, the introduction to the CSA recognizes the possible medical benefits of controlled substances, many of which "have a useful and legitimate medical purpose and are necessary to maintain the health and general welfare of the American people." The issue for Raich and Monson's defense is not only the medical benefits of controlled substances, but marijuana's Schedule I classification and the overarching importance of protecting the "health and general welfare of the American people."[19]

These cases set the stage for subsequent decisions that moved the question of medical marijuana closer to its current state, which is illustrated most clearly in *U.S. v. Oakland Cannabis Buyers' Cooperative* (2001). California's 1996 Compassionate Use Act provided ill patients with the legal ability to acquire and use marijuana for medical purposes. The Oakland Cannabis Buyers' Cooperative (OCBC) was organized for the purposes of cultivating and providing medical marijuana under the law, with a staff that included a supervising physician and registered nurses. Membership required written documentation from a physician and successful completion of a screening interview. The federal government sued the cooperative for violation of the CSA. The district court placed a temporary injunction on OCBC's activities, which the cooperative ignored, continuing its operation. The district court ultimately rejected OCBC's defense after determining none of the users were in danger of imminent harm.[20]

OCBC argued that the distribution of marijuana was medically necessary because only it could alleviate its patients' pain. OCBC advocated either dismissal or a "medical necessity modification" to the federal injunction. In his rejection of OCBC's appeal to medical necessity, district court judge Charles Breyer adapted standards established in *U.S. v. Aguilar* for a medical necessity defense, namely:

(1) the patient suffers from a serious medical condition; (2) if the patient does not have access to cannabis, the patient will suffer imminent harm; (3) cannabis is necessary for the treatment of the patient's medical condition or cannabis will alleviate the medical condition or symptoms associated with it; (4) there is no legal alternative to cannabis for the effective treatment of the patient's medical condition because the patient has tried other legal alternatives to cannabis and has found them ineffective in treating his or her condition or has found that such alternatives result in intolerable side effects.[21]

Judge Breyer found that OCBC patients did not meet these standards. At the same time, the standards themselves are riddled by layers of evaluative criteria. George Annas notes that federal standards do not bestow medical necessity upon treatments that are as good as other available treatments, but require "scientific evidence showing that marijuana [is] better than other approved drugs for any specific medical condition."[22] The CSA, moreover, does not recognize cost as a consideration. Seizing upon these openings, and accepting physicians' determinations about the imminence of harm and lack of legal remedies for the conditions marijuana was used to address, the Ninth Circuit Court of Appeals reversed the district court's decision.

In 2001 the Supreme Court voted unanimously to overturn the lower court and argued that the CSA does not allow a medical necessity exception *even if evidence could be mustered to establish its legitimacy*. According to the opinion, the CSA only allows for possession for government approved research projects, and "the defense cannot succeed when the legislature itself has made a 'determination of values.'"[23] The nuances of the court's reasoning are instructive. Justice Stevens, in a concurrence, agreed with the majority that the CSA prohibits a medical necessity defense, but took issue with the court's questioning of medical necessity defenses in general, as "the Court gratuitously casts doubt on 'whether necessity can ever be a defense' to any federal statute that does not explicitly provide for it, calling such a defense into question by a misleading reference to its existence as an 'open question.'"[24]

The turn to the language of "value" instead of evidence is worth pausing on. Federal standards do not consider treatments that are as good as other available treatments to be medically necessary, but require "scientific evidence showing that marijuana [is] better than other approved drugs for any specific medical condition."[25] In other words, the CSA's handling of marijuana is rooted in an empirical claim about marijuana's efficacy compared to other options, but also hinges its classifications on available evidence. This is important because the exploration of marijuana's biomedical uses is hindered by the CSA itself, which makes it difficult to study marijuana's potential benefits in a rigorous manner. While the federal government has allowed some trials to take place under specially-approved programs, marijuana lacks the kind of critical mass of clinical data that other remedies have been able to accumulate, regardless of whether they are deemed effective. In 2015, a Brookings study noted, "Statutory, regulatory, bureaucratic, and cultural barriers have paralyzed science and threatened the integrity of research freedom in this area," adding that "moving marijuana from Schedule I to Schedule II would signal to the medical community that FDA and NIH are ready to take medical marijuana research seriously, and help overcome a government-sponsored chilling effect on research that manifests in direct and indirect ways."[26] Paradoxically, the argument that medical marijuana lacks clinical evidence is in large part a function of the self-fulfilling prophecy of federal scheduling itself. The value of medical necessity must remain largely unknown under these conditions.

On one hand, therefore, there is a question of what to make of more than thirty states legalizing medical marijuana, and almost a dozen legalizing recreational marijuana, despite marijuana's federal classification under the CSA. There are few such glaring examples of direct conflicts between federal and state laws. On the other hand is a more prescriptive question of where medical necessity determinations, backed by the force of law, are best made. For example, in their study based on a three-prong test for determining as a threshold matter whether the federal government should assert preemptive jurisdiction over the policy, Pickerill and Chen found that policies regarding medical marijuana are best left to the states.[27]

At the same time, of course, while there can be a legitimate debate about the proper role of governance within a federal system, ultimately the question of medical marijuana is one of the substance's safety and effectiveness, which is a matter for biomedical science to determine and for regulators—especially the FDA—to approve and oversee. To understand how government has reconciled itself with this tension, I now turn to some of the strategies with which both federal and state governments have managed the problems created by the CSA scheduling. The result is less a resolution of the central problem—marijuana's scientific basis within the politics of medical necessity—than a political compromise to mitigate the effects of a stringent, and seemingly intractable, legal standard.

Medical Necessity Defenses

The legal context created by the CSA and congressional resistance to revisiting the scheduling of marijuana has created a situation in which the medical use of marijuana is carried out through a series of exceptions to the law. It is here that the politics of marijuana and the legal context of necessity intersect and clash. These exceptions include allowing medical necessity defenses and sentencing mitigation for violation of state laws, and federal tolerance of state laws in contravention of the CSA through federal deprioritization policies.

Before turning to legal medical necessity defenses within the context of the politics of medically necessary marijuana, some general comments about medical necessity defenses are in order. Specifically, legal readings of medical necessity must consider such defense's longstanding history rooted in common-law notions of necessity itself, which are the foundations of American legal defenses, and of direct consequence to medical necessity. The celebrated English jurist William Blackstone summarized these as follows:

> Both the life and limbs of a man are of such high value, in the estimation of the law of England, that it pardons even homicide if committed *se defendendo*, or in order to preserve them. For whatever is done by a man, to save either life or member, is looked upon as done upon the highest necessity and compulsion. Therefore if a man through fear of death or mayhem is prevailed upon to execute a deed, or do any other legal act; these, though accompanied with all other the requisite solemnities, are totally void in law, if forced upon him by a well-grounded apprehension of losing his life, or even his limbs, in case of his non-compliance.[28]

Admittedly, "death or mayhem" is a high bar. But it is important to notice that necessity establishes a qualitative boundary. Others would set it differently.

The rhetoric of necessity manifest as legal force arises prominently in the so-called necessity defense, famously evoked in the 1884 British case of *Regina v. Dudley & Stephens*. In that case, three shipwrecked sailors opted to eat a forth sailor, a seventeen-year-old boy. Despite their arguing that they had no choice but to sacrifice one to save three, the court found them guilty of murder, noting that there was no clear necessity since they could have been rescued at any moment (as they eventually were, though it is not clear that they would have all survived had they not eaten the boy).[29] Blackstone argued as well that such defenses could also apply to misdemeanors. In *Scott v. Shepherd*, for example, a man threw an explosive into a market, which was subsequently tossed around by merchants and eventually exploded and blew a man's eye out. The first man was held liable while the self-preservation acts of the other merchants were found to not constitute malicious or criminal intent. It is important to notice, however, that Blackstone acknowledges a range of exceptions—not just death—in his view of necessity. Accordingly, "The right of personal security consists in a person's legal and uninterrupted enjoyment of his life, his limbs, his body, his health, and his reputation."[30]

Of course, medical necessity defenses are not the same as necessity defenses in general. But they help us to get closer to understanding the "necessity" in medical necessity. The stories that support these defenses are often marginal and challenging. For example, an Ohio man evoked a medical necessity defense to explain why he crashed his car into and injured three people.[31] According to the driver, a diabetic condition suddenly impeded his ability to control the car. This position conjures the more well-known necessity defense utilized in cases in which a norm is claimed to have been breached not by choice, but because the agent responded to a set of unavoidable conditions. Borrowing from Aristotle, necessity can be a defense to the extent that it establishes that an action was not a choice—suggesting that if it were a choice, the agent would have chosen otherwise.[32]

Medical Necessity Defenses in Marijuana Cases

Some legal scholars argue that since there is an injustice in denying marijuana to those who could benefit from its possible medical uses, American courts should allow a medical necessity defense that acknowledges that some people, in an attempt to get themselves what they need to survive and reduce pain, are justified in breaking federal law. There is some precedent for this. Recall that, in his concurrence in *Oakland Cannabis Buyers Collective*, Justice Stevens reasserted the existence of a common-law defense of necessity, "even in the context of federal criminal statutes that do not provide for it in so many words."[33] This raises a question not only about when and under which conditions medical necessity defenses are valid, but, more precisely, when they are recognized as such. Pongratz argues, "The medical necessity defense should be available as a relevant excuse or justification of violations of CSA provisions dealing with use and/or possession of marijuana, on the ground that medical need renders the violation of the CSA the lesser of two evils."[34] To be sure, the medical necessity defense does constitute a potential compromise, but it amounts to an approach in which reprieve is provided by courts, not through legislative action. Justice is proffered through exceptions.

The case of William Kurtz illustrates how legal options change the landscape of extralegal medical necessity defenses. Kurtz, a sixty-two-year-old native of Washington State, has spastic paraplegia, also known as Strumpell-Lorrain disease, which affects the optic nerve, causes epilepsy, cognitive impairment, peripheral neuropathy, and deafness. Physicians can only offer symptom management, and conventional treatment for this condition does not exist. Police arrested Kurtz in 2010 after discovering forty-two marijuana plants, for which Kurtz lacked proper authorization such as a medical marijuana card. Though prosecutors could not establish intent to sell, the state of Washington charged him for growing and possessing marijuana. At the time of the 2010 trial, the judge did not permit the use of a medical necessity defense precisely because state-issued cards were available, even if not easy to secure. The court found him guilty, fining him $4,000 but no jail time. On appeal, however, the state supreme court sided with Kurtz, noting that prosecution should not be the preferred approach for "those few people who fall through the cracks and haven't complied by crossing their T's and dotting their I's as to the medical marijuana act." Nonetheless, the judges disagreed as to the broader legal context. Signaling a shifting legal terrain, one judge noted in dissent, "Because individuals in this state have a legal way of using medical marijuana, the previously articulated common-law defense of medical necessity for marijuana use is no longer appropriate."[35]

Kurtz's case can be fruitfully contrasted with that of Cathy Jordan, a Florida woman with amyotrophic lateral sclerosis (ALS), commonly known as Lou Gehrig's disease. In February 2013, police raided Jordan's house on suspicion of marijuana possession after a real estate agent showing a house next door reported seeing Jordan's plants. Believing that she met all qualifications of a medical necessity defense, her partner Robert Jordan kept detailed records of her use, as well as reactions to each use. Upon learning that Jordan had ALS, prosecutors dropped all charges. As he left the courthouse, Robert noted, "We were doing this for 16 years and you know now finally it went through the legal system and they're saying that we're right all along. I've been saying that there is no pharmaceutical can do what the plant does."[36] Jordan's lawyer added, "When a woman tells you she's outlived four or five of her support groups, let her continue treatment."[37] The couple continues to lobby for marijuana legalization. Cases such as Jordan's suggest the possibility that medical necessity holds special meaning for those with complex needs or debilitating disease. Should there be a different standard of medical necessity decision making for those in such situations? Should medical necessity be complexity dependent? Should the seriousness or dire state of a patient's health alter how we think about medical necessity and, for present purposes, the degree of risk that a medical professional may justifiably take in violating the law?

This dilemma puts some medical professionals in a difficult spot. This is especially true for pharmacists. For example, given the tensions in federal and state laws, it is unlikely that pharmacists could successfully evoke a medical necessity defense if they act in what they perceive to be patients' best interests. At the same time, while physicians may recommend marijuana, it is pharmacists who are charged with the important role in American medicine of ensuring patient safety with regard to medications. Because of CSA scheduling, pharmacists are largely cut out of the quality control process, leaving a question about who, if anyone, oversees the safety of marijuana being sold in various states.[38] CSA scheduling means that the FDA does not oversee the production, distribution, or sale of marijuana, which means that the quality and safety of medical marijuana is largely unknown, unpredictable, and hard to assess.

Medical exemptions to the CSA on the federal level have come slowly. While not an undoing of the CSA, or a change in the scheduling of marijuana, the most significant sweeping development to date came in 2009 when Attorney General Eric Holder announced that "it will not be a priority to use federal resources to prosecute patients with serious illnesses or their caregivers who are complying with state laws on medical marijuana, but we will not tolerate drug traffickers who hide behind claims of compliance with state law to mask activities that are clearly illegal."[39] In other words, while neither decriminalization nor a formal legislative development, the deprioritization of marijuana prosecution affords states considerable space in which to work. Such space, of course, depends upon political outcomes, as the next presidential administration could reverse the order with little trouble. Many medical marijuana advocates hope that deprioritization is a first step toward the rescheduling of marijuana. At the same time, President Donald Trump's first attorney general, Jeff Sessions, made clear his intention to crack down on marijuana possession, including in states that have legalized medical or recreation use. According to the Trump administration, these efforts will not make medical marijuana distributors and users a priority, though it is unclear how they will distinguish between these different justifications. While this is a rollback from the Obama administration's directives, Congress has thus far refused to fund special programs designed to enforce the CSA.[40] The result is a continual lack of clarity within both the medical and recreational marijuana industries in more than a dozen states. Among other things, failure to resolve tensions between the CSA and state law, as well as accommodate

studies that would shore up the evidence base for marijuana's medical benefits, has created a set of conditions in which both the legal and medical
structures lack clarity. This lack of clarity has tremendous consequences for
long-term health care planning, especially for patients with chronic conditions, hinders the much-needed and careful study of the benefits and risks
of marijuana in clinical contexts, and creates legal uncertainty that is not
productive from either a health outcomes or policy perspective.

Necessity defenses, with the attendant sentencing mitigation they can
license, are promising strategies for softening the edges of a contradictory
legal code within a tiered federal system. Their efficacy, however, is uneven
within federal systems. The key variable within the American context is
state law, with some states having legalized or relaxed penalties for possession, or becoming more open to sentencing mitigating in response to
medical defense arguments or expressed needs. Other states, however, continue to enforce strict and even imperious laws. Perhaps the best known
is the case of Lee Carroll Brooker, a seventy-five-year-old disabled veteran
in Alabama who experiences chronic pain. After a 2011 arrest Brooker was
sentenced under Alabama law, which mandates that people with prior
felony convictions who are found to possess more than one kilogram of
marijuana are to be sentenced to life in prison without a possibility of pa-
role.[41] In 2016, the U.S. Supreme Court refused to intervene in Brooker's
case, in which Brooker had argued that his sentence was a violation of
the Eighth Amendment's prohibition of cruel and unusual punishment.

As my discussion of medical necessity, in general, and medical marijuana, in particular, makes clear, the lack of clear legal standards is a key
problem for the politics of medical marijuana. At the same time, as should
also be clear by now, legal clarity is unlikely to resolve the thorny issues
raised by marijuana policy debates precisely because medical marijuana's
legal contexts are bound up in nonlegal discourses ranging from the biomedical to the political. I next examine the relationship between medical
marijuana and regulatory mechanisms on the federal and state levels.

Federal and State Regulation and Medical Necessity

The American federal system adds another layer of complexity, especially considering the wide programmatic and regulatory variation that
exists from state to state. This lack of uniformity across states becomes
particularly pronounced in debates about medical marijuana. Conceptu-

ally, the differences in health care policy accomplish what early American thinkers thought states were well positioned to accomplish, namely the idea that states could serve as laboratories for policy approaches that other states could either mimic or reject. The result, however, is rhetorical dissonance, as the coexistence of competing and contradictory jurisdictions and degrees of illegality and criminality makes it clear that the question of marijuana is not merely one of legitimate medical usage, but an inherently political question.

The interplay between federal and state oversight is a critical part of the broader political dynamic. While the vast majority of medical necessity regulation remains on the state level, a function of states' traditional police powers of health, safety, and general welfare as generally assumed under the Tenth Amendment of the Constitution, there are also notable stopgap measures, often issued in the name of antidiscrimination protections in which the unwillingness of providers to cover certain procedures is challenged by federal mandates. As we would expect of American political culture, there is significant resistance to the establishment of federal medical necessity standards at the same time as certain procedures and modalities of care (especially expensive ones) are attended to.

Both federal and state law play crucial roles in regulating medical necessity. The Center for Medicare and Medicaid Services explains:

> The mandatory home health services benefit under the Medicaid program includes coverage of medical supplies, equipment, and appliances suitable for use in the home. . . . A State may establish reasonable standards, consistent with the objectives of the Medicaid statute, for determining the extent of such coverage . . . based on such criteria as medical necessity or utilization control. . . . In doing so, a State must ensure that the amount, duration, and scope of coverage are reasonably sufficient to achieve the purpose of the service [and] may not impose arbitrary limitations on mandatory services, such as home health services, based solely on diagnosis, type of illness, or condition.[42]

Such guidelines directly affect medical necessity determinations. Consider, for example, a decision that held that Arizona, despite the recommendation of its health care cost containment system, could not refuse to cover incontinence briefs. The specific reasoning is instructive, as the judge rejected Arizona's argument that "absent some condition that mandates the briefs, like a rash, nothing in the law requires taxpayers to fund them." The judge rejected the state's argument not only that these items were expensive, but that requiring one service necessarily forces cuts to others. According to the judge, Arizona "cannot unilaterally decide what services it can afford."[43]

Some critics who prefer the establishment of federal standards lament the flexibility afforded state governments and insurance providers in determining and overseeing medical necessity decision making under the ACA. The consequences of leaving medical necessity open to state interpretation are most acute with regard to the potential for discrimination.[44] For example, benefits that do not specify the means by which benefits can be accessed may leave women worse off than they were, or at least in a less predictable situation. Indeed, there is a great deal of difference in states' medical necessity frameworks and appeals processes, especially under Medicaid, as some states explicitly include cost considerations while others exceed minimum coverage requirements to include that which others consider elective, hence not strictly necessary.[45] Critics uncomfortable with the vicissitudes of state politics generally prefer to see the ACA's benefits extend not only to abstract essential benefits, but to the provision of actually accessible care at the point of delivery.

These preliminary comments on federalism lay the groundwork to illustrate how medical marijuana laws are handled. Not only do state laws differ, and sometimes wildly, but "this confusion is exacerbated by the level of variance in types of medical marijuana legislation supported by different medical, professional and policy advocate groups."[46] Legal and rhetorical dissonance follows as state laws fall into three quite different categories: type of provision, illnesses and symptoms covered, and supply of marijuana. With regard to the first category, moreover, Pacula and colleagues identify at least four distinct ways states statutorily enable the medical use of marijuana, each of which creates unique tensions with federal law: therapeutic research programs, rescheduling laws, physician prescription laws, and medical necessity defense laws, underscoring the wide range of approaches available to states, from proactive arguments about therapeutic benefit to legal defenses.

The story, of course, is more complicated than federal supremacy. The various competing legal standards and jurisdictions also constitute distinct rhetorical domains that underpin the political dimensions of medical marijuana debates. Federal law, after all, stands in tension with the opinions of many medical experts and physicians, as well as laws that allow for the regulated distribution of marijuana for medical purposes.[47] The continual appearance of state ballot initiatives reminds us that these arguments are in progress and persistent, as the medical necessity of marijuana seeks to penetrate the power/knowledge cluster that sustains current law. These insurgent movements are not only medical, scientific, and legal, but political as well. As such, they make clear that federal intransigence on the matter of CSA scheduling is only partially related to the state of scientific consensus over marijuana's medical benefits. Indeed, they are caught up in stakeholding, lobbying, and other forms power.

Physician Authority and the Legitimation of Medical Marijuana

Medical marijuana debates tend to center on the potential benefits for patients, as perhaps they should. However, the politics of marijuana and medical necessity have consequences for medical professionals as well. If "legitimate" marijuana harvests are inherently questionable, so are marijuana prescriptions. If patients are subject to suspicions of moral hazard when marijuana is widely available through sometimes suspect routes, even if they lay claim to being medical, the judgments of physicians and other medical professionals who sanctify that legitimization should be similarly suspect. The AMA's position on medical marijuana reflects this dynamic insofar as it is designed to defend physicians against prosecution rather than legitimize a medical treatment.[48] This position is unsurprising considering the AMA's primary role in protecting physicians, but it also underscores the difference between the rhetorics of patient-centeredness and professional autonomy. They may be related and reinforcing, but they may also work against one another.

More commonly, arguments opposing the current federal scheduling of marijuana take a two-pronged approach, pointing to potential patient benefits as well as the importance of respecting physician determinations. Many advocates of medical marijuana have appealed to physicians' authority and expertise in attempting to distinguish legitimate from illegitimate use. Some state laws reflect this. For example, the California Compassionate Use Act not only evokes the relief that marijuana can provide to patients, affirming the existence of the benefits that the CSA denies, but cites instances in which "medical use is deemed appropriate and has been recommended by a physician who has determined that the person's health would benefit from the use of marijuana."[49] The California act evokes physicians' authority as a hedge against federal prosecution, pitting physician determinations against those of the federal government.

Accordingly, an important part of the medical marijuana literature centers not only on physician–patient relations, but physicians' broader social and professional legitimacy.[50] This makes sense since state laws passed in defiance of the CSA utilize physician prescriptions as primary justifications. The legitimacy of prescriptions, of course, is grounded in an assumption that physicians have adhered to professional standards, grounding determinations in professionally sanctioned medical need instead of patients' recreational preferences. Yet, it should also be said that physicians must remain credible actors for this dynamic to hold, since medically necessary marijuana is rooted in physicians' professional judgment, and is therefore a function of their credibility and ethos, both of which are critical components of rhetorical effectiveness. To this extent, the distinction between recreational and medical marijuana depends not upon a medical standard, but upon professional legitimacy and legitimation through behaviors.

Recall that *Raich* attempted, unsuccessfully, to use physicians as a rhetorical counterweight to the CSA. Specifically, the decision held that the advice of a physician cannot be construed as sufficient evidence to contradict the CSA's position that marijuana has no known acceptable medical uses.[51] In considering the consequences of this congressional determination, as well, it is important to consider the tradition of off-label uses for approved drugs, by which physicians are allowed to prescribe for uses other than those specifically identified by FDA approval. Drugs that are not included in Schedule I are afforded physician discretion while Schedule I substances are excluded from uses within the broader category of the medical in general.

The question of physicians' roles in medical necessity decision making regarding marijuana was not decided by *Raich*, however. Two cases, *U.S. v. Aguilar-Ayala* (1997), heard in the U.S. Court of Appeals for the Ninth Circuit, and *Conant v. Walters* (2000), decided by the U.S. District Court for the Northern District of California, affirmed the right of physicians to recommend medical marijuana, even though they could not lawfully prescribe it. To this extent, American law is composed of tensions between patient needs and physician autonomy, on the one hand, and state and federal law, on the other.[52]

We can learn a great deal about physicians' roles in these debates by noticing how physicians are situated rhetorically within state legal contexts. Some states call for a determination made by one physician for a marijuana prescription, while others require two. Beyond the number of physicians who approve, some states call for new and often close scrutiny of physicians, with severe penalties (beyond those of other forms of prescription abuse) in the event that recreational marijuana is found to have been prescribed under the cover of medical justification. In other words, medical marijuana debates are entwined not only within a changing politics of marijuana, but ongoing developments in the role that physicians play in broader power structures in American society itself.

Policing the Boundaries of the Medical and Recreational

Beyond the legal contexts within which marijuana is situated are a series of boundary questions that frame the larger politics of medical marijuana. The rhetorical basis of these questions tends to center on slippage between medical and recreational use. To grasp the nature of the contests that shape this boundary, therefore, we must consider explicit challenges as well as the subtler movement that tends to occur between the medical and recreational.

Conjuring necessity's Aristotelian roots, one common complaint is that states that have legalized marijuana for medical purposes have made it too easy to procure, raising the specter that the medical justification, purportedly driven by clinical judgment, is in fact a cover for recreation. Beyond lax laws that appear to have been written to relax these boundaries is a concern, once again, about moral hazard, in which porous boundaries between the medical and the recreational create opportunities for those individuals who abuse the law. Contributing to this mythos, a myriad of media reports set out to show that securing required documentation such as a medical marijuana card is easy, the suggestion being that holders of these cards do not have, in many instances, legitimate medical need. A San Diego news station claimed, for example, that many medical marijuana cards amount to "get out of jail free cards" and are misused. The report quotes a dispensary worker who argues that abuse doesn't undermine the existence of medically necessary marijuana, but "hurts our cause and the people we are truly trying to help."[53]

Other reports focus on questionable practices by dispensaries tasked with guarding the legitimacy of medical marijuana. One, for example, seeks to undermine this legitimacy by emphasizing the ubiquity of dispensaries, noting that that there are more marijuana shops than Starbucks in Los Angeles, where the scope of availability is portrayed as outpacing reasonable conceptions of possibly legitimate medical need. According to one community member quoted in the story, the result is an "Alice in Wonderland circus" leaving communities, presumably aggrieved by the proliferation of the shops, with little recourse: "People here are desperate, and there's nothing they can do."[54] Adding to the suggestion that medical marijuana laws serve as cover for otherwise random and often illegitimate access to marijuana, another article describes a competition between the author and his wife, the former with "writer's cramp" and the latter with rheumatoid arthritis, to see who could access a medical marijuana card. The former succeeded while the latter, whose physicians would only sign for advanced cases of cancer, failed.[55]

While most of these problems are due to the logistics and credibility of medical marijuana dispensaries themselves, these problems also raise questions about what kind of delivery systems, financial arrangements, and public accommodations should be made available to support medical marijuana. These criticisms take aim at the related infrastructure and accommodation rather than marijuana itself. In each case, as particular contexts are filled out, medical marijuana's legitimacy is threatened. In 2013, for example, as Illinois's Compassionate Use of Medical Cannabis Pilot Program Act was set to be enacted, a discussion about implementation occurred in the Naperville city council, where a councilmember asked, "Is there a medical necessity to have a drive-thru? If there's a solid rationale, from a medical standpoint, I'd like to know."[56]

Similarly, in Wisconsin, a representative of a local chapter of the National Organization for the Reform of Marijuana Laws appealed to Republican objectors by arguing that they should embrace medical marijuana as part of the governor's jobs program, presumably because medical marijuana would—as it has in other states—create a new economy. The proposed (though ultimately failed) law that the representative was addressing would have created a medical necessity defense for those who wished to prove medical need. But the Wisconsin case illustrates the complicated nature of such debates. Senator Leah Vukmir, chair of the Wisconsin state senate Committee on Health and Human Services and an opponent of the bill, challenged the medical framing of the issue, noting, "What I resent most is this façade you are putting forth, using people who are dying of cancer, using people who have other illnesses, as your shield, and I think it's something more than a ruse for you to move towards full legalization of marijuana," adding, "I wish you would come right out and admit that."[57] Depending on one's perspective, Vukmir's skepticism could be read as a rejection of the medical or a defense of an outwardly political framing of the marijuana question.

These examples illustrate a unique feature of medical necessity marijuana debates. Whereas the boundaries between medical necessity and the cosmetic and the experimental, or even social necessity, tend to characterize most medical necessity debates, blurred boundaries between the recreational and the medical play a central role in the politics of medical necessity and marijuana. At issue in this distinction is the familiar question of whether the rhetoric of necessity is being deployed in situations that are, in fact, choices. Unlike the cosmetic versus medical distinction, which is often accompanied by an association with need (especially as concerns employability and other forms of social acceptance, which in turn can be linked with health) recreation denotes enjoyment. Cosmetic surgery also includes reconstructive needs following injuries related to fire or war, which evoke widespread sympathy. Cosmetic care does not necessarily reduce to the vain celebrity sort, but often addresses actual and serious concerns, regardless of whether various entities within the politics of medical necessity, including payers such as state and federal taxpayers or insurance companies, agree. Marijuana's connection to discourses of liberty and recreation set it apart from other arguments used to frame medical necessity debates since discourses of recreation cannot be stretched to necessity and, in fact, tend to serve as a polar opposite. Accordingly, as we have seen with legal standards, medical necessity discourses are tethered to need and even desperation.

A different set of arguments arise when marijuana debates eschew medical justification and openly advocate recreational use. These arguments connect with a theme I have evoked throughout this book, namely the epistemic clarity that can come from openly political debates, which has the additional benefit of enhancing the integrity of legitimately medical questions. Many of these arguments are purely pragmatic and economic, such as those that concede to marijuana's inevitable proliferation but seek to capitalize—quite literally—on the situation.

Political culture plays a role as well. An article in the *Economist* argues, for example, that these ballot initiatives would have the effect of making marijuana available "without the sop to puritanism of medical necessity," focusing instead on "the ills of prohibition and the economic benefits of legalization."[58] Accordingly, this marks a direct and open engagement with the politics of medical necessity. Dispensaries operating in the name of medical necessity, but suspected to be fronts for illegal, nonmedical marijuana sales, have the effect of undermining the idea of medical necessity itself. In this sense, the current politics of marijuana in the United States pits advocates of recreational marijuana against advocates of medical marijuana, with potential damage to the principled rhetorical bases of both causes. Federal regulations that force marijuana to travel under the sign of medical necessity undermine the ability of medical necessity itself to remain useful for the regulation of medical care. Specifically, medical marijuana needs the integrity that can be purchased only through rhetorical distance from the rhetoric of recreation.

As with most medical necessity arguments, however, the distinction between recreational and medical use of marijuana falls into liminal spaces instead of tidy analytic categories. Calls for legalization are, in one sense, calls for allowing for a more honest marijuana discourse, grounded in the political rhetoric of freedom rather than need. Such a grounding preserves not just the discourse of medical marijuana, but the medical generally. Nonmedical legal marijuana use allows marijuana users to speak openly rather than through proxy discourses demanded by the law. Similarly, it would seem that clarity regarding the boundaries between marijuana's medical and political justifications would be important to those law enforcement and public health officials who oppose legalization. It would also clarify the matter of funding, where recreation would not raise political and social questions about public goods, while medical marijuana might command necessary social resources.

Though the strategy of waging marijuana battles within the discursive field of medicine may be successful in the short term, marijuana's long-term medical value requires, at a minimum, a revision of the categories that shape the rhetorical debates that stymie more critical thinking. The present moment is a critical one for this revision, for two reasons. First, there is a matter of the medical itself, as marijuana's benefits accrue not usually to patients' physical healing or cure, but the alleviation of pain, comfort, and the redress of ancillary effects of treatment itself. In this regard, the medical necessity of marijuana can be said to remain on the margins of the medical, related to but not quite medicine. The fact that marijuana's benefits tend to be secondary changes the way risk must be assessed, but also pushes us to think anew about the importance of palliation and comfort in health care. Second, recent developments underscore the extent to which medical marijuana debates interact with traditionally nonmedical political arguments, which means that a political question is at issue. Specifically, those who seek to use medical arguments to secure access for recreational use are both failing to engage politically, insofar as politics requires a modicum of openness about one's position, while making the lives of those who seek legitimate medical use significantly more difficult, forcing them to operate under a specter of fraud. This specter is particularly acute when ascertaining what we might somewhat awkwardly call the "medicalness" of something that has long been cast as a source of joy and relaxation instead of palliation or cure.

In a sense, those who make recreational arguments under the guise of medicine cannot be blamed. In theaters of contentious politics, political actors commonly utilize the rhetorical tools that are available to them. As Peter Cohen notes, "in the absence of federal evaluation and regulation, individual states have taken the initiative in legalizing the medical use of marijuana. In doing so, however, they have created what is essentially a regulatory vacuum."[59] Cohen argues, "Inadequately crafted and enforced regulations should not allow misguided and inappropriate claims of medical necessity to act as a subterfuge for the de facto legalization of 'recreational marijuana.'"[60] The crucial point is that the situation created by current law essentially makes the ethical and fiduciary responsibilities of physicians the foundation of legitimate medical marijuana. This is a lot to ask of physicians.

What is needed is a sustained critique not only of medical discourses, but of how depoliticizing forces tend to put medical discourses in the position of having to do the work that political argument should. In other words, the prevalence of medical necessity arguments and defenses can be read as a symptom of civic decline not only with consequences for medicine, but politics. Recent developments suggest a possible opening. Ballot initiatives have played a major role in the legalization, on the state level, of both medical and recreational marijuana. While ballot initiatives and bills passed through traditional legislative processes have provoked consider-able debate about effects, especially disagreements about the impact of the new laws on "drugged driving"[61] and accidental ingestion among children and pets due to the proliferation of edibles,[62] they also appear to be reshuf-fling the political decks, since marijuana need not travel under the sign of the medical in these states. In other words, one important feature of state-level developments in recreational marijuana laws was that they addressed the problem of false medical necessity. While one can (and should) de-bate the merits of recreational and medical marijuana, the presence of two categories does release considerable pressure from the medical. Along the way, it both frees and returns integrity to the rhetoric that sustains medical marijuana itself.

Medical necessity tends to arise as a binary rhetoric of necessary or not. But this means that the medical is only meaningful insofar as it can be juxtaposed with that which it is not—and is therefore dependent on a structural, if fictive, "other." While permissive recreational marijuana laws may raise questions for public health and law enforcement, the main bene-ficiary of their arrival may be the legitimation of marijuana laws arising in purely medical contexts. This is not to say that the boundaries will not con-tinue to be stretched and contested. Instead, medical necessity will no lon-ger have to do all of the political work asked of it when it serves as a proxy for those who seek nonmedical marijuana. This political move has impor-tant consequences not only for medical marijuana, which, in some states that have both, is now distinct from recreational uses, but for the medical itself. If trends continue, the most important epistemic difference between medical and recreational marijuana is likely one of financing, as insurance providers and governments decide whether to accept the medical justifi-cations for paying for medical marijuana. Blurring of these categories and fraudulent claims will, of course, continue to be an issue. But compara-tively concrete analytic categories will help to sort out disagreements.

This chapter has emphasized three critical dimensions of medical mari-juana's relevance to the politics of medical necessity. First, considering marijuana's widespread use as a recreational drug, this analysis provides an opportunity for rethinking the boundaries of its medical legitimacy in relation to its nonmedical uses. This is important considering the skepti-cism medical marijuana evokes in those who oppose the liberalization of marijuana laws, on the one hand, and opportunism vis-à-vis the medical by those who support such liberalization, on the other. Second, the existence of the rhetorical spheres of recreation and medicine creates a politics in and of itself, with consequences for the further and deeper understanding of boundary drawing between medical and political rhetoric insofar as they shape manifestations of power/knowledge. Third, the case of medical marijuana helps us to think more clearly about tensions between medicine and the law. The shifting terrain, with some states passing medical marijuana laws and others legalizing recreational marijuana, illuminates the relationship between medically-sanctioned treatments and a stubborn federal legal approach that leaves the carving out of exceptions, as medical necessity defenses, as the only option in many cases. Within the broader politics of medical necessity, the case of marijuana illustrates the role that long and seemingly intractable histories can have on constraining our ability to think clearly about the scope of medicine, and medicine's role within the political. But what happens when we move from a deficit in our knowledge of a plant's effects on the body to an expansive universe of conditions that are not only not always inscribed on the body in an observable manner, but which also must be witnessed through the observation of behaviors and through speech?

4

Contesting the Medical Necessity for Mental Health

In May 2017, the National Alliance on Mental Illness, a prominent national advocacy organization that agitates in support of rights of the mentally ill, rallied in support of expanded mental health services in Iowa. The group marched in support of proposed bills that would increase funds for bed capacity for mental health patients in the area's hospitals, and to force Iowa's three managed care organizations to pay providers in a timely manner, streamline preauthorization procedures, and standardize insurers' use of the term "medical necessity."

Though the bills did not pass, the march is representative of similar mobilization that occurs from time to time around the country. It is also illustrative of the key challenges that mental and behavioral health advocates face in the United States, as well as their significance for the politics of medical necessity. This march put on display the intertwined problems associated with defining medical necessity, the precarious status of mental and behavioral health as a matter of insurance provision, and the political place of mental health advocates vis-à-vis insurers and other stakeholders in American health care. As the bills' sponsor noted at the march, "Preauthorization is taking so long and many times it's rejected, so the patient may be sent home without the patient getting the test the doctor thinks they need."[1] Advocates called for the establishment of more rigorous medical necessity standards as one way to combat discrimination directed toward those dealing with mental and behavioral health problems.

It seemed smart to address medical necessity directly. After all, as the psychiatrist Daniel Knoepflmacher has argued, "Without universal medical necessity criteria for mental health care, clinicians and their patients are saddled with a concept highly susceptible to abuse by insurers. For now, multiple class-action suits are the main fronts in the battle against restrictive coverage criteria that limit access to appropriate psychiatric care."[2] However, as Knoepflmacher acknowledges, such an approach is suboptimal in terms of the interests of patients. It is also a largely unsustainable strategy, as contesting medical necessity one lawsuit at a time is not only inefficient, but an unpredictable foundation on which to build an enduring and reliable approach toward medical necessity.

Despite the inefficiencies and inequities that depending on lawsuits poses for medical necessity decision making, there is good reason to hope that a focused legal strategy could move us closer to establishing such standards. The cases where mental health needs are rejected in the name of medical necessity are many, and each case is potentially serious to the individual whose declared need, even if confirmed by a clinician, is rejected. Despite policy developments promising parity between mental health and physical health conditions, it is nonetheless the case that many Americans struggling with addiction and other behavioral health needs continue to fight with insurance companies, who often issue rejections in the name of insufficient medical necessity, and at a rate that many perceive as disproportionately targeted at mental and behavioral health needs.[3] The gains that have been made in federal and state law with regard to mental health are promising. Yet resistance to applying new standards fully and fairly suggests that stigma about mental and behavioral health, disbelief regarding the legitimacy of mental health diagnoses, and concern over increased costs continue to fester. The persistence of these problems is an effect of the politics of medical necessity itself.

Compounding the definitional issues associated with medical necessity is the historical fact that the domain of mental and behavioral health has long endured attacks on its legitimacy.[4] Mental health is shaped by some of the dynamics I have reviewed in previous chapters, while adding qualitatively and politically different dimensions to our understanding of medical necessity. To unpack these dynamics, this chapter contains three parts. First, I examine the rhetorical moves at work in mental health medical necessity, with a particular focus on how political debates about medicalization in mental health intersect with mental health coding regimes. Second, I offer a reading of a widely cited article on the subject of medical necessity and mental health: a now more than two-decades-old essay by James Sabin and Norman Daniels entitled "Determining 'Medical Necessity' in Mental Health Practice."[5] This essay not only illustrates the critical fault lines in mental health medical necessity debates, but serves as a useful snapshot of a changing terrain, written at the height of scholarly and political debates about the ethical and medical consequences of managed care, but before passage of the Mental Health Parity and Addiction Equity

Act (MHPAEA) in 2008 and subsequent developments in this history. Third, and subsequently, I examine how the terrain that has developed in the years since the publication of Sabin and Daniels's piece compares to the landscape that served as their backdrop. Here I describe the present state of mental health debates in light of the broader politics of medical necessity, especially mental health parity debates.

The specific touchpoints that distinguish the time when Sabin and Daniels wrote their piece and the present are the passage of the MHPAEA, the reaffirmation of mental health parity in the ACA in 2009, and the publication of the fifth edition of the *Diagnostic and Statistical Manual of Mental Disorders* (DSM-5) in 2013. These threads of the current politics of mental health constitute relatively new spaces for thinking about medical necessity as a practical instead of merely technical tool of medical and health care rhetoric, a tool that different clinicians and advocates of mental health can and must determine how they wish to relate to. The decisions that confront clinicians and advocates are important even as medical necessity in mental health remains a critical, and flexible, appellation for those patients trying to secure care that they need at the margins of American social and political culture. To this extent, the politics of medical necessity in mental health are part of shifts taking place in the broader legitimization of mental health as a standard piece of broader health conversations.

Medicalization and Mental Health

I briefly raised the question of medicalization in earlier chapters to emphasize the extent to which such debates call into question the very meaning of what does and does not qualify as medical. I also emphasized that medicalization is not merely a category mistake (though it may sometimes be), or a merely stigmatizing label called upon to pathologize social problems (though it may also sometime be this too),[6] but is often the price for accessing important treatments and modes of care for patients whose conditions would not otherwise be recognized. This, as should be clear by now, is a result of the special rhetorical force that medical discourse has in American health care debates.

A well-known recent example is the medicalization of the needs of transgender Americans, who in many cases needed to subsume themselves in the psychological discourse of Gender Dysphoria, codified in the current version of the DSM, to gain access to various forms of care.

While I do not review the politics of transgender health in depth here, it is instructive for thinking through the dynamics of medicalization within debates about gender identity. Patients and advocates are understandably split on the medicalization of transgender needs, with some concerned about the stigma that may accompany this move and the loss of other narratives, such as bodily autonomy and freedom, while others emphasize the care that DSM codification can enable and the doors that it can open.[7] In most cases, advocates of more robust medical and health care services for transgender people must recognize that the turn to the medical frame will always be mixed. In some—even many—cases the specter of suicidality and other forms of self-harm, as well as violence generally, frames mental health justifications for medical necessity declarations for sex reassignment surgery and hormone therapy.[8] The rejection of important health care services that transgender people may need to live flourishing lives may, paradoxically, create new dangers that fall within the purview of mental health.

What is clear is that the role medical necessity plays in mediating these relations has both a repressive as well as a productive potential. The history of mental health service provision has long been concerned with this persistent double-edged sword. After all, while the pursuit of a life in which one can flourish may not appear to individuals as a medical consideration, such a framing may be the most effective or even the only means available for securing care within existing health care regimes. The intersection of gender identity and need is also always at risk of raising the specter of disorder from those tasked with governing an existing power/knowledge regime, as we have seen in recent years in restrictive bathroom laws.[9] Yet negotiating these regimes, governed as they often are by cisgendered, heterodominant systems of power, may be a person's only chance of accessing care or important services. In these situations, medical necessity's gatekeeper role—and the medicalization it carries with it—can constrain individuals' ability to be truthful about who they are in order to make themselves socially legible. In health care discourses, medicalized bodies become legible bodies capable of being subsumed and codified within medical and other systems. The same is true, in the arena of mental health, with the mind. It is for this reason that those who fall outside the binary structure of necessary-unnecessary must often seek positions of social legibility from within the medical order to gain recognition. They must recast themselves within a recognizable language of medicine. It is therefore important that political projects concerned with securing access to care utilize whatever tools may be available to aid people in need. Yet, such projects should turn to these tools in full awareness of potential shortcomings and even traps that those tools may possess.

Understanding why much of the growing literature on medicalization has developed in the area of mental health is key to understanding what is unique about its intersection with medical necessity. According to Thomas Szasz, perhaps the best-known critic of the medicalization of mental health, new diseases such as hysteria come about not because new phenomena are discovered, but because "the criteria of what constitutes disease have been changed—from the psychochemical derangement of the body to the disability and suffering of the person."[10] Accordingly, a range of conditions—"hysteria, hypochondriasis, obsessions, compulsions, depression, schizophrenia, psychopathy, homosexuality—all these and many others thus became diseases."[11] Others have echoed Szasz's sentiment. Medical sociologists Peter Conrad and Valerie Leiter argue, for example, that the application of the antidepressant drug Paxil to anxiety disorders "has contributed to the medicalization of emotions, expanding medical jurisdiction over emotions such as worry and shyness."[12] Allen Frances, a DSM critic and prominent skeptic about the medicalization of mental health, sees far-reaching consequences of the trend. Specifically, he links the stigmatization that comes with labeling those with psychological challenges as "mentally ill" with the prescribing of "unnecessary, harmful medications, the narrowing of horizons, misallocation of medical resources, and draining of the budgets of families and the nation."[13]

The perspectives brought to bear by these critics should remind us that the prefix "medical" in medical necessity often functions doubly. Those seeking care must establish that their condition is medical—that is, for strategic reasons they must medicalize their condition or participate in an existing medical discourse—to secure services. At the same time, those attempting to assert independence may resist medicalization with the goal of keeping medical regimes and their accompanying modes of social control at bay. Of course, companies that stand to gain from marketing medical solutions for problems that were previously regarded as nonmedical are all too happy to embrace increased medicalization. A great deal of effort by the billion-dollar medical industry, including the pharmaceutical lobby, is concerned with establishing the medical legitimacy of various products and services. The DSM has long been the central front in the war over classification, and some critics regard the move from the third edition of 1952 to the fifth edition of 2013 as a shift from psychology to psychiatry, which largely tracks the movement from talk therapy to pharmacology.[14] Insofar as "classification systems . . . emerge from the crucible of human experience," the classification of mental illness has emerged in large part from the experiences of war and social strife.[15] Psychiatry's legitimation of the medical model is a response to social maladies with cultural, political, and policy implications. As such, it carries with it the potential for social control.

Despite many patients' complex relationships with medicalization, the debate itself is also, as we should expect in the Foucauldian register, double-edged, and must be read with this in mind. On the one hand, it is important to police the boundaries of medicalization, not only because those boundaries have serious ethical consequences for how we care for and treat people, as well as the subject positions medicalization's disciplinary practices create, but also how it drives health expenditures that can put pressure on and even undermine systems. On the other hand, the skepticism calls into question the motivations of those who may be the only ones capable of mobilizing resources for people in need. Indeed, as the previous chapter showed in the case of medical marijuana, the general skepticism about institutional determinations has eroded the usefulness of the classification of diseases itself. The result has been a tendency on the part of some critics to undermine and poke fun at these new conditions rather than engage in a critique of conditions that arise as societies develop and decline.

The introduction of new disorders meets predictable cultural resistance, especially from critics of overdiagnosis and overmedication. This is especially the case along lines of certain target populations, such as at the intersections of race, gender, class, and sexuality.[16] For example, girls are two-thirds less likely to receive a clinical diagnosis of attention deficit hyperactivity disorder (ADHD) than boys, although this difference disappears by adolescence.[17] Oppositional defiant disorder (ODD), an illness related to behavior seen as disruptive, is also significantly more likely to be diagnosed in boys.[18] That boys are more likely to be diagnosed with ADHD and ODD likely has roots in a gendered form of social power and socialization.

Clinical approaches to ADHD medical necessity decision making are also often racialized. A widely cited 1999 study of Baltimore's public schools found that ADHD diagnoses were dramatically more common among minorities and low-SES (socioeconomic status) children. Yet, controlling for economic status and gender, the study found that ADHD medications were prescribed twice as often to white students than to minorities. The authors of the study reported: "It is possible that ADHD is more prevalent in low-SES and minority populations than in higher-SES and nonminority populations, and that the observed differences reflect parents' decisions to fill prescriptions and/or to make prescribed medication available to their children in school."[19] The study noted that previous research found that African American youths were prescribed stimulants less often than white youths.[20] There is a lack of hard data on why these gaps in prescription and diagnosis exist, but it stands that in the case of ADHD, there is a marked racial difference in medical necessity determination.

In addition, people of lower socioeconomic status are more likely to be diagnosed with a multitude of mental disorders, although there remains a debate regarding whether socioeconomic status causes mental illness or individuals become poor as a result of their symptoms.[21] There is compelling evidence that we remain in the midst of the ongoing medicalization of poverty, which has the corollary effect of obscuring the role played by environmental factors.[22]

A critical reading of the development of mental health classifications reminds us that the politics of medical necessity is one of conceptual and rhetorical invention, and not a mere linear recording of empirical facts. Compounding this observation are critiques by experts in the field that resist the medicalization of mental phenomena that have been absorbed into medical models over the past decades.[23] At the center of this question is the political economy of an American pharmaceutical industry that has commodified medical knowledge to such an extent as to place it under persistent doubt, which is fueled in large part by the powerful force of direct-to-consumer marketing. The industry's marketing tactics, in turn, fuel patients' anxieties and push them to self-diagnose.[24] Compounding critiques of profit motives, as well, is a persistent critique of the role the FDA has played as a regulator—a role that often appears to be captured by the very industry it is charged with overseeing.[25]

In terms of medicalization, I follow Casper and Clarke's approach, which "assumes that 'rightness' and 'wrongness' are socially constructed, partial, and contingent."[26] The belief—perhaps sometimes true, but other times clearly not—that a mental health condition is unobservable causes a problem for medical necessity, which thrives on the observable. At a minimum, mental health opens doors for rhetorical debates that would not be as appropriate, for example, in gastroenterology or cardiology. However, to the extent that this distinction between observable and nonobservable medical necessity holds, the medicalization of somatic conditions is more easily conceptualized than the domain of mental health. But this, it must be noted, is only because of historical pathways in which health was focused on bodies, often at the expense of mental and behavioral considerations that have only in recent decades started to be taken seriously by clinical professionals, researchers, and health care institutions. Accordingly, in the realm of mental and behavioral health, as recent history has approached the matter, the conceptualization of disease can include conditions bounded only by the limits of human experience, strife, and suffering. These maladies and needs therefore appear to require more extensive conceptualization, revelation through conversation and self-report, and other strategies that do not sit easily alongside the history of somatic health conditions. Insofar as we may seek to medicalize mental health complaints to gain access to insurance coverage, therefore, we are necessarily entering a domain characterized by a degree of subjectivity, but one that becomes increasingly important to value. We should therefore expect to find—and do find—that these debates would be even more contentious than those addressing the coverage for medically necessary surgery or other physical interventions. To illustrate the properties of this interpretative domain, I now turn to a reading of common rhetorical moves in mental health medical necessity debates.

Rereading Sabin and Daniels

Sabin and Daniels offer a theoretical framework for medical necessity decision making in mental health. These boundaries acknowledge that medical necessity is not merely a clinical question, but a marker of "moral disagreement."[27] Their review, which draws on six real-life examples from the Harvard Community Health Plan, yields three models for categorizing medical necessity in mental health. Each model is tested for what they consider to be an important difference between "treatment" and "enhancement," the latter of which exceeds the common clinical understanding of medical necessity. They distinguish, as well, between what they call "hardline" and "expansive" clinicians.

Each of Sabin and Daniels's cases illustrates a challenge posed by boundaries. At the same time, in watching them navigate these divisions we observe critical rhetorical moves within the politics of medical necessity. For example, they describe the situation of a patient, called Shy Bipolar, as "fully analogous" to somatic conditions such heart failure, diabetes, or lupus, "which require ongoing outpatient medication management, and which most standard insurance plans cover." In justifying this case vis-à-vis traditional medical interventions, Sabin and Daniels note, "Insofar as the case management focuses on dysfunctions that arise from the bipolar illness, such as monitoring moods or coping with demoralization, the appointments are analogous to advice regarding exercise and nutrition for a patient with cardiac disease or diabetes."[28] The epistemology of illness that Sabin and Daniels advance is formulated in large part by aligning various conditions to create a robust picture of mental illness in relation to somatic conditions.

Of particular interest for understanding mental health's location within medical necessity discussions is the need to analogize mental health to the medical model. Such an understanding illuminates the extent to which insurance coverage for mental health relies upon persuasive strategies to secure mental health's legitimacy as a medical question that is in turn afforded conceptual parity with physical medical needs. This association of the medical model with mental health underscores the extent to which increased social understanding of mental health appears to have not shaped medicine itself, for example by expanding our understanding of the goals of health care. Instead, mental health advocates have sought to find a place for mental health within existing classificatory structures.

As we should expect, however, in some cases the analogy does not hold. After all, as Phyllis Foxworth, vice president of advocacy for the Depression and Bipolar Support Alliance, has noted, "Medical necessity is a big, dark hole around mental health parity."[29] In ways that individuals with somatic pain would rarely be dismissed, the patient labeled Cranky Victim, who experienced deep unhappiness in his life, was found to be "maladaptive" but not "inflexible," suggesting that his request for individual instead of group therapy was unfounded and medically unnecessary. For Sabin and Daniels, this inflexibility suggests that Cranky Victim is responsible for his situation, which pushes against the typical justification for medical necessity in marginal cases. But Sabin and Daniels add a twist, evoking the possibility, perhaps through genomic research, that Cranky Victim's situation could one day be found to have a genetic basis, which could potentially change the rhetorical structure of his situation.

Leaving aside the question of genetics and medical necessity (to which I return in the conclusion), for now it must suffice to address the question of choice and agency. Sabin and Daniels compare Cranky Victim's case with that of another patient, Lost Administrator, a woman with myriad interpersonal problems and diagnosed with atypical depression, under the care of the same clinician. In considering the two cases, the clinician admitted that "he felt decidedly more sympathy for the Lost Administrator than for the Cranky Victim and worried about how his reactions may have influenced his reasoning about medical necessity." Moreover, he remained uncertain as to whether his diagnoses "explained his judgment of medical necessity, or whether he had invoked [DSM] diagnoses to justify his moral assessment that the Lost Administrator 'deserved' treatment" while the Cranky Victim did not.[30] It is not only the role that judgment plays that is significant in these cases, but the evocation of moral and political categories such as responsibility and deservedness.

In another case, a woman (Abandoned Mother) did not meet DSM criteria for depression, but her symptoms suggested the need for some kind of intervention, which she received in the form of outpatient therapy. Sabin and Daniels note the difficulty with ambiguity:

> The concept of medical necessity forces us to pose questions in an either-or manner: treatment is or is not medically necessary. Clinical situations like the Abandoned Mother's, however, are often much more ambiguous. Further observations may help but do not always take away the uncertainty.[31]

Since, in the abstract, medical necessity is ambiguous, it is incapable in and of itself of resolving unclear situations in medical necessity decision making. In the case of Abandoned Mother, subsequent discussions yielded an increase in her "suicidal preoccupations" such that she was afforded weekly case management. Here the existential possibility of suicide appears to have clarified an otherwise ambiguous situation.

According to Sabin and Daniels, insurers' concern with expanding medical necessity's scope in mental health centers on the problem of moral hazard, which I have evoked in earlier chapters. The unique properties of mental health diagnosis make the specter of moral hazard uniquely concerning, particularly insofar as symptoms of mental illness are "part of a continuum with everyday forms of distress," making many diagnoses "controversial and uncertain." In addition, they argue that treatments, including psychotherapy, can appear "similar to nonprofessional forms of human support and interaction."[32] This raises concern about offering limitless coverage in a policy domain characterized by scarcity, and people's willingness to pay out of pocket is construed as a kind of test of the real need. When people really need something, the suggestion goes, they will find a way. Accordingly, UnitedHealthcare's overview of its handling of medical necessity notes that though "services rendered that are deemed NOT medically necessary during pre-service review will not be covered," members "may choose to move forward with service which will result in member liability."[33]

Sabin and Daniels respond to these challenges with three models for reasoning through difficult cases: normal function, capability, and welfare. Normal function accepts inequality in the distribution of human capabilities as something that health care cannot change, at least on a large scale. The capability model sets as a goal the mitigation of differences in human capabilities and devotes more generous resources to the most disadvantaged, thereby requiring a more expansive understanding of medical necessity toward those ends. The welfare model approaches wellbeing (and medical necessity) most expansively, operating largely outside of formal mental health diagnostics, especially the DSM. Taken together, the three models form a continuum in which the availability of insurance coverage for mental health services becomes increasingly expansive. Sabin and Daniels advocate the normal function model, which they believe the public and clinicians will regard as fair, can be administered "in the real world," and is affordable. They argue that this model allows for the drawing of a "plausible boundary" with which to govern insurance coverage.

Tellingly, Sabin and Daniels make clear that not only the vicissitudes of judgment, but public opinion and support play a critical role in establishing these criteria. This is because "historically tenuous" support for mental health coverage must be protected—not only, or even primarily, in terms of clinical rigor, but in public perception and support. The goal here is to retain the system's perceived legitimacy and avoid pushback. This is particularly important as concerns public health programs in which the expansiveness of mental health services under Medicaid, Medicare, and other services may rise and fall with the public's sense that medical necessity is being constructed narrowly, thereby closely policing moral hazard.

Sabin and Daniels also illustrate some of the rhetorical tensions in the broader politics of mental health medical necessity. They hold, for example, that medical necessity is not only a clinical question, but a signal of "moral disagreement,"[34] a point that seems particularly important for mental health. This moral disagreement, it is worth noting, directly bears on the relationship between medical power and knowledge. The political categories that continually arise in Sabin and Daniels's article—judgment, public perception, legitimacy, and scarcity—underscore the political nature of the question. Attentiveness to the expansive lexicon in play in mental health discussions serves as a rhetorical reminder that medical questions are always located at the intersection of social power.

Mental Health Parity and Medical Necessity

In 2009, when the ACA was passed and Americans began to understand its contents, the inroads the bill made in moving the American health care system toward parity in services for mental and behavioral health provoked considerable if not unsurprising backlash. At issue was a question of tremendous rhetorical and political significance, namely whether mental health was analogous to physical health. The secondary and practical significance of this question was whether mental health could fit into the same financing paradigms, and could be rooted in similar evidence bases, as somatic conditions. Building on the MHPAEA, the ACA's mental health parity provisions require that individual and small group coverage for mental health and substance abuse be generally comparable to coverage for medical care.

While these slices of the broader insurance terrain may seem small when compared to the larger group market and government health plans, the ACA's reaffirmation of these parity provisions was intended to close important gaps by mandating that all plans sold on ACA marketplaces provide mental health and addiction services. There is little question that these provisions advance the cause of bridging historical gaps between access to care for somatic conditions and mental and behavioral health needs. Marking a shift in philosophical as well as policy-level commitment, the ACA provides support for training behavioral health care providers to increase access and improve disparities.[35] The infusion of new monies into mental health in existing and new health centers could reduce stigma surrounding mental health and addiction, and increase the number of facilities proximate to high need areas, particularly in rural and urban areas.[36] These parity provisions are a key piece of the medical necessity puzzle.

Beyond the still-elusive question of defining medical necessity in mental health practice, Sabin and Daniels were prophetic about the reaction that ACA parity debates would have. Because of a belief that mental health is less precise than other aspects of medicine, or that patients and clinicians may abuse medical necessity's vagueness, insurance administrators often "fear that if mental health services were given parity with other medical services . . . insurance funds will be siphoned into a 'bottomless pit.'"[37] The ACA's parity provisions excited many advocates of an expansive view of mental health medical necessity. Others have concerns, however. For example, though insurance companies had to fund mental health services, they "retained the right to determine whether sessions were 'medically necessary,'" which they did by requiring utilization reviews that appear to have been intensified post-ACA.[38] The price of parity, in other words, appears to be stricter controls on the terms of discourse regulating access, with medical necessity placed at the center. The lack of a clear definition of medical necessity—even by consensus—is compounded by the powerful gatekeeper role it is ascribed within insurance processes.

According to psychologist Darcy Lockman, who reports increased frustration in working within insurance companies post-ACA, insurance companies appear to be playing rhetorical games not only with medical necessity, but other important gatekeeper concepts as well. For example, Lockman reports that insurance companies deploy a too-restrictive use of the word "crisis," as well, which in mental health is of extreme importance, especially with patients contemplating suicide. In such situations, insurance company recognition of the existence of a crisis, or validation of a clinician's declaration of such a state, is paramount for establishing medical necessity. Lockman concludes that "'crisis,' like 'medical necessity,' is whatever the insurance company says it is in order to justify not paying."[39] Fewer crises, of course, result in cost savings within the politics of medical necessity, underscoring the rhetorical structure of urgency that underpins the rhetoric of medical necessity. While this dynamic existed to some degree in the early post-ACA years, when cost concerns remained comparatively low, parity provisions intensified in 2014 when the bill was fully implemented and more Americans were insured. The perceived need for tighter controls appears to have been a major driver. At this time, in

Lockman's experience, insurers' dependency on utilization processes intensified. But this process lacked a strong will to enforce as well as a clear standard for oversight.

This general unenforceability mirrored the ACA's approach, or lack of approach, to medical necessity itself, which undermined some of the gains in mental and behavioral health. Thus, while the MHPAEA required that health insurers publish their medical necessity criteria,[40] scholars have noted that both the MHPAEA and ACA codified insurers' discretion in developing processes for determining medical necessity. This is not unusual considering how federal legislation tends to handle medical necessity. For example, Title XIX of the Social Security Act, which governs Medicaid, holds that while states may not deny benefits on the sole basis of "diagnosis, type of illness, or condition," they "may place appropriate limits on a service based on such criteria as medical necessity."[41]

While provisions such as those that govern public and private plans may suggest the presence of some barriers to discrimination, the openness of the language concerns some scholars. Suann Kessler argues, however, that the specific language of the MHPAEA and ACA "empowered" insurers to "pick and choose which mental illnesses to cover."[42] Lacking clear standards that could serve as the basis for patient access to services, the ACA's approach to medical necessity for mental health was only as strong as the level of advocacy that came to support it, through appeals and publicity. As readers will recall, this dynamic mirrors the early development of medical necessity itself in the 1970s, which moved from a tool to secure access to a mechanism for encoding unpredictability, at a minimum, or—even worse—restricting it. This suggests an important axiom for the politics of medical necessity in mental health. Specifically, medical necessity, with its ability to narrow and constrain the scope and nature of care, may be the key tool that insurers use to evade government mandates that excite clinicians and patients. Paradoxically, recent parity provisions have intensified the politics of medical necessity as it appears in mental health insurance provisions.

Beyond objections to subjecting patients and their clinicians to elusive medical necessity standards, mental health sits uncomfortably within the politics of medical necessity because of the very nature of the kind of symptoms and diagnoses it addresses. At the center of this discomfort is what one legislator who sponsored the MHPAEA calls "outdated distinctions between disorders in the brain and illnesses in the body."[43] This question returns us to a more traditional conceptualization of the body within the politics of medical necessity, a conceptualization that pits bodies against minds. Evoking the insurance industry's concern with increasing costs, a representative of America's Health Insurance Plans noted, "A treatment plan for diabetes or a chronic heart disease is very different from a treatment plan for a patient that's seeking care for depression or another mental illness." In a revealing addendum, the representative noted, "It's not a math formula,"[44] with the apparent suggestion that physical health interventions can be reduced to such formulas in ways that mental health cannot. Similarly, a former CEO of Magellan Health and Maryland Mental Health Director noted that mental health professionals "can micromanage care down to almost nothing," adding that "enforcement in this area is a joke."[45] The assumption, it seems, is that medical necessity can be juryrigged and even faked in ways that supposedly observable physical health cannot. Yet, this seems to miss the important fact that all health—physical as well as mental—exists on a continuum of observability. In making these distinctions, critics seem to be linking the observable with the objective, which in turn becomes tethered to medical necessity discourses. Yet, considering the power afforded medical necessity in American health care, the consequences of carving up the epistemic world of medicine in this way has grave consequences not only for mental health, but for the place of primary care, preventive health care, and wellness. In other words, the preoccupation with objectivity and specificity appear to be concerned with maintaining a regime of power/knowledge that, in turn, privileges more conventional views of medicine.

Many mental health advocates view parity provisions as a critical step toward a more balanced understanding of medicine's aims, especially concerning the conceptualization of the body and mind. These include some members of the insurance industry, such as a Cigna CEO who noted, "Disconnecting the mind and the body, which is the way historically insurance wanted this, doesn't make any sense."[46] For others, however, this raises a pragmatic question of measurement. Sheila Schuster of the Kentucky Psychological Association, asks, "On the physical health side, you've got blood pressure readings and X-rays. But how do you measure the depth of someone's depression?"[47] Similarly, T. M. Luhrmann notes the challenge of identifying problems in psychiatry, as well, noting,

> There are no diagnostic tests in psychiatry. . . . You cannot draw someone's blood, stick someone in a magnetic resonance imager, or take any medical reading that will tell you definitively whether that person is depressed or not.[48]

Of course, many efforts do exist to standardize the measurement of depression, notably psychiatrist Aaron Beck's well-regarded and widely used 1972 depression inventory, which takes seriously individuals' self-reporting about their condition, and uses that self-report to garner medical legitimacy.[49] As is the case with any widely used and respected measurement tool, the Beck Depression Inventory is constantly being rethought and updated, especially with regard to concerns about its applicability across cultures and potential—though as yet unsubstantiated—racial bias.[50] Efforts are also underway to ensure that the Beck inventory correlates with revisions to the DSM. The Beck inventory, above all, seeks to lend structure to understanding how to link patients' conditions in a rigorous manner to the very preconditions—the description of needs—that underpin medical necessity decision making. In turn, the inventory serves as an important tool for ensuring that mental and behavioral health needs are taken seriously, and are well positioned to interact with more familiar, longstanding measurement tools used in health care. In so doing, the Beck inventory, and others like it, constitute an important step toward legitimizing mental and behavioral health needs within biomedical models.

As we have seen with the needs that advocates claim medical marijuana addresses, symptoms rooted in physical conditions are in many ways no less difficult to address than those that exist in mental health. As gender theorists and others have shown, social contexts shape the phenomenology of bodies, as well as medical diagnosis and treatment.[51] The boundary between the physical and mental does not reduce the complexity of medical necessity's interpretative dimensions. On the other hand, stigma in mental health medical necessity decision making appears to be due in part to its lack of the kind of visible, material grounding that medical necessity's conceptual gatekeepers demand of both diagnoses and outcomes. Recent investments in mental health resources appear to be largely due not to a fundamental change in conceptions of the medical, but a function of the widespread media attention that American soldiers have received, especially with regard to post-traumatic stress disorder. Similarly, whether founded or not, the attention that advocates of relaxed gun laws have focused on mental health may have the result of increasing public resources, even as they may increase the biased view that violence is a function of mental health instead of weak controls on access to guns. The difficulty is seeing medical necessity through the often-dense thicket of social and political controversy that frequently accompanies issues such as guns, abortion, marijuana, and the like. Thus, precisely where Szasz saw physical conditions as more straightforward than conditions of mental health— where there were "clear-cut bodily diseases such as syphilis, tuberculosis, typhoid fever, cancer, heart failure, and fractures and other injuries"[52]—a careful reading of medical necessity shows bodily need to be just as subjective, just as socially laden, and just as open to debate.

The slow development of mental health's legitimacy vis-à-vis biomedicine has been at the center of its politics. The struggle for the legitimacy that would even allow mental health to participate in the rhetoric of medical necessity has come at sometimes high costs. Although preliminary discussions leading up to the introduction of the DSM-5 generated widespread skepticism and even jokes—notably for its proposed "internet addiction" disorder,[53] but other proposed classifications as well—the historical development of mental health is one of increased, if slow-to-come, legitimacy. This movement is due in large part to the persistent efforts of patient advocates and key professional organizations, but also as the social impact of mental health epidemics becomes increasingly pronounced and known. This appeal for legitimacy has been difficult because the DSM had previously medicalized issues that were, in hindsight and after much agitation, revealed to be grounded not in clinical judgment, but bias and discrimination. The medicalization—and subsequent demedicalization—of homosexuality is well known and has been studied extensively.[54] But it is important to remember that that story is just one of many.[55]

It is important to remember, as these examples illustrate, that new clinical criteria must always tarry with history, as well as the systems of power/knowledge that function within and arise from within that history. Medicine has to overcome past errors made and social biases imported into the diagnostic categories that comprise its historical development. Perhaps the most notable development in this field is the increased social acceptance of and concern for post-traumatic stress disorder, once largely dismissed and consistently stigmatized, but now considered a central clinical classification for victims of violence, military personnel, and other trauma sufferers. As with many dimensions of the epistemology of medical decision making, what comes to be accepted as medically necessary is always, more or less, a function of social power. This is perhaps truer in the arena of mental health than any other.

These conceptual differences are critical to debates about mental health parity, where they serve as foundations for policy making. The power of the MHPAEA is its requirement that both group and qualifying individual insurance plans' "financial requirements and treatment limitations on Mental Health or Substance Use Disorder benefits . . . are no more restrictive than those on medical or surgical benefits."[56] These requirements are critical because mental health and addiction are, despite some progress in combating stigmatizing trends, often treated as moral failures, lapses of personal responsibility, or, at an extreme, insidious medicalization strategies to pathologize otherwise common life struggles. To this extent, parity critics are sometimes concerned that the price—the medicalization of mental health—is too high.

One option is removing mental health from the medical model altogether and viewing it as raising an altogether different set of questions. Greenberg, one prominent critic of the DSM whose work represents this position, notes, "no one knows what would happen if psychiatrists simply let themselves out of their epistemic prison [of the medical model] by no longer pretending to know what they can't know."[57] For Greenberg, the risk to psychiatry's legitimacy that would come from eschewing the medical model is worth the risk because of the impact it could have for caring for patients: "By no longer insisting that it is just like the rest of medicine, and by renouncing its noble lies about the scientific status of psychiatric diagnosis, the profession might become a more honest one than it is now."[58] Such a move would allow for an entirely different set of rhetorical practices to accompany discussions about mental health. In the interest of serving patients better and more honestly, Greenberg recommends that we define a mental disorder as an instance of "suffering that a society devotes resources to relieving."[59] But here again we note the problem with this definition, as the acknowledgment of social values, absent a mandate to finance care, leaves social resources unsecured. This unpredictability, of course, could have grave consequences for those in need. Given the institutional and political economic systems in place in American health care, we should not be sanguine about the prospects.

In light of the limitations of this approach, it is worth exploring others. Health insurance providers, for example, may be convinced to embrace expansive medical necessity arguments if so doing minimizes long-term costs that would stem from the need for more extensive and expensive medical care in the future.[60] In this view, behavioral and mental health would benefit from an evidence base showing more completely how it contributes to total patient care, which could in turn be lodged in a broader picture that includes overall cost savings in the longer term. For example, denying outpatient psychotherapy to someone may be shortsighted if that person ends up hospitalized for major depression. Short term resistance to declaring treatment medically necessary may not only fail to help—and could even hurt—patients, but could also end up costing more in the long run.

This more expansive approach to medical necessity—even one that challenges conventional intuitions about the meaning of the term—may be justifiable and even persuasive in the long run. It may provide benefits to patients and payers. Precisely where parity raises concerns among payers who are skeptical of mental health's objective grounding and wish to narrow the meaning of "medical" to exclude prevention and wellness, one can envision opportunities for benefiting from medical necessity's interpretive flexibility. From this perspective, this could license early care that would likely have been rejected in order to avoid later, far costlier care. The intersection of mental health and medical necessity sends us back to the politics of medical necessity itself, where a pliable, less fixed discourse becomes a useful site for contestation and advocacy.

5

Reproductive Politics

The Cases of C-Section and Abortion

It is unsurprising that the conceptualization of bodies would play a central and often fraught role in the politics of medical necessity. After all, the fact that bodies are physically observable in no way minimizes their interpretability. Health needs and medical judgments are always bound up in rhetorical structures that give them their social character. At the same time, it is also the case that certain aspects of bodies receive more attention than others, and certain bodies—especially those of sexual and racial minorities, and women—are part of a particularly contentious politics. This too should be unsurprising. After all, as Foucault once noted, these intersections, especially those that involve sexuality, constitute "regions where the grid is tightest, where the black squares are most numerous."[1] Medical necessity debates often, if not always, center on questions of what Cindy Patton calls "medico-moral *techne*" concerning matters of sexual identity, and the role that power plays in regulating gender norms, sexuality, and reproduction.[2] Despite the predictable contentiousness of these questions, it is important to understand how the interaction between clinical decision making and the politics of medical necessity that we have examined is refracted through the categories that police bodies.

This chapter explores the intersection of reproduction and medical necessity by examining two distinct but, as we shall see, interrelated topics: abortion and C-section. Abortion and C-section are, of course, united in their grouping under the broader rubric of reproduction and women's health. They are distinct, however, to the extent to which one is concerned with terminating a pregnancy while the other is a means of carrying out the delivery of a baby. As I shall argue, it is the collective value of these similarities and differences that makes it useful to examine C-section and abortion together. To document the unique political and clinical contexts in which we find these different aspects of women's health, I first evaluate each on its own before offering readers an opportunity to consider them together. This approach is intended to give due attention to the unique political and rhetorical placement of abortion and C-section within medical necessity debates before attempting to ascertain what light an analysis of both abortion and C-section together might shed on them.

Cesarean Section

I have argued that the misguided presumption that an objective grounding exists in medical necessity discourses often gives rise to some of medical necessity's most politically important and rhetorically interesting dimensions. It is therefore unsurprising that a similar dynamic exists when engaging the question of whether C-section is medically necessary. The hope in the case of C-section, as with medical necessity generally, is that there is or could be clear guidelines that would make the decision purely clinical, outside of the disciplinary effects of social power, and grounded in medical fact instead of persuasion. Yet, given the complexity involved in circumscribing the medical, especially as it operates rhetorically within the context of reproductive politics, the decision to deliver by C-section is far more complicated than these epistemic assumptions suggest.

Before turning to C-section, however, some comments on the history of the medicalization of childbirth are in order. After all, as in the other areas I have examined, it is in the theater of medicalization that the politics of C-section, as well as abortion, take place. Central to this history is the fact that the well-documented rise and legitimation of the AMA was made possible in large part by the medicalization of childbirth, a move made simultaneously with the delegitimation of midwifery.[3] The AMA was founded in 1848 to unite physicians' organizations, but did so in large part by sidelining nonphysician "irregulars" from delivering babies. Among their goals were requiring physicians to attend college and establishing new medical standards and licensing laws that would prohibit midwives from playing a significant role in childbirth. In so doing, the organization defined the medical in an explicitly gendered manner, building physician authority atop a recognition that "midwives were an easy competitive target for medicine."[4]

The rhetorical warrant for replacing midwives with newly certified physicians was safety, not professional privilege, despite the fact that outcomes between medicalized delivery and midwifery were comparable.[5] This reminds us that navigating the politics of medical necessity in C-section debates requires getting clear on the benefits of legitimate medical progress as opposed to the social forces—sexism, professional positioning, financial opportunism—that drive other aspects of C-section debates. Beyond the observation that an organization of increasingly powerful male physicians seized upon childbirth for professional gain, the idea that women could both give birth and attend to birth became unthinkable. Giving birth became "the quintessential feminine act."[6]

The role that gender plays in the epistemic structuring of childbirth, with consequences for how C-section is understood, was confirmed by a recent study that found that women often frame their thinking about childbirth "in terms of the tensions they navigate concerning their feminine bodies as heteronormative sites of pleasure and sexuality on one hand and sources of endless, selfless maternal nurturance on the other."[7] Many women in this study did not cast their preferences regarding C-section or vaginal delivery in purely medical terms, but instead evoked a rhetoric located more broadly at the intersection of gender and sexuality, as further evidence that considerations of medical necessity and childbirth are bound up in the preservation of cultural norms and may be read as clear functions of social power and the knowledge to which it is bound.[8] Considering the power of these social narratives, compounded by the physician perspectives I have explored above, patient perspectives are highly conditioned and constrained, their rhetoric generated largely if not (at times) completely from widely circulating discourses. This claim of a physician's right to circumscribe and define, and ultimately control the medical "gradually gave to doctors the medical control of birth."[9] To this extent, rising C-section rates in the United States suggest the need not only for questioning their medical necessity, but for asking what role specifically gendered power and gendered rhetoric played in the establishment of these histories. This both challenges the simplistic appeal to the rhetoric of choice and serves as evidence of the power/knowledge arrangements that shape how women, as well as other supporting actors, view C-section.

The decision to deliver by C-section is no mere alternative to vaginal delivery, but a decision of consequence and qualitative distinction. C-section is a major surgery requiring large abdominal incisions, regional and sometimes general anesthesia, and a two- to three-day hospitalization. C-section, moreover, does not evade the risks of vaginal delivery, but introduces complications of its own, including higher rates of hemorrhage and blood clotting, the need for transfusions, risk of infection, and increased postpartum depression.[10] One study found mortality rates for babies born by C-section, absent other complications, to be more than double that of vaginal delivery.[11] Studies have also documented wide regional variation in the likelihood of delivering by C-section, suggesting that geography skews perceived medical necessity.[12] While C-sections may reduce some contingencies and complications stemming from labor, they may also introduce infection and error, with different effects—as we would expect—along class and racial lines.[13] For example, Lisa Ikemoto argues that nonwhite and poor pregnant women are more likely to be forced into medical treatment than their more affluent, white counterparts. According to Ikemoto, resistance to such forced treatment gives rise to an enduring and racialized stereotype:

> She has little education. Perhaps she does not understand the nature of her refusal to consent. She is unsophisticated, easily influenced by simple religious dogma. She is pregnant because of promiscuity and irresponsibility. She is hostile to authority even though the state has good intentions. She is unreliable. She is ignorant and foreign. She does not know what is best. The cases ascribe these characteristics to the bad mother; this is the subtext, the things that can nearly be said. They make it easier to assume that the woman's will should be overridden. They also offer moral grounds for intervention. The expressions of anger, frustration, and righteousness in the case reports and opinions strongly evoke the things that can nearly be said. Not stated is that these assumed characteristics are particular to stereotypes of poor women of color. So, what goes unsaid is that she is Black; she is Hispanic; she is Asian; and she is poor.[14]

Appealing to medical necessity to justify C-section is a serious and not uncomplicated matter, with particularly serious consequences for women of color, who are more susceptible to stereotyping by health care workers.

Since changes in C-section rates are contextual, we need to understand how underlying historical conditions inflect perception of the surgery's medical necessity. As medical historian Jacqueline Wolf explains, during the 1940s and 1950s, C-section rates rose from "negligible to measurable," at about 2.5 percent of births. This number was largely a function of "medically justifiable reasons," that converted C-section, previously an extremely dangerous last resort, into an increasingly successful—though still risky—procedure.[15] Among the developments that made C-section a more viable option in situations of extreme medical emergency was the invention of anesthesia.

American women originally received C-sections primarily to deal with breech births, or births in which the baby is not positioned for head-first delivery. While 11.6 percent of such births were carried out by C-section in 1970, by 1984 that number had reached 80 percent,[16] 85 percent by 2003,[17] and—in at least one national sampling—94.8 percent by 2015.[18] Though physicians are often assumed to be a driving force in rising C-section rates, the real story is more complicated. In fact, evidence suggests that most physicians do not mention or advocate for C-section when a patient is not thought to be at risk of breech delivery.[19] Instead, most decisions appear to be functions of what are often billed as women's preferences, themselves shaped, of course, by various aspects of a gendered, economically-inflected social power. Yet, here this narrative is again too simple. Many critics, for example, have cast doubt on the clinical validity of physicians' support for so-called maternal request C-sections because C-sections benefit physicians financially. That such procedures evoke a rhetoric of being "on-demand" conjures the charged rhetoric of "abortion-on-demand" as well as the familiar concern regarding perceived moral hazard based purely on patient insistence that is so often entwined with medical necessity debates.[20]

Some critics suggest that at least some physicians may steer patients toward C-sections because they are less disruptive to schedules,[21] reducing them to a decision of convenience instead of necessity.[22] Yet the move to payment reforms emphasizing value and outcomes, instead of fee-for-service models in which clinicians are paid for services performed, could have a positive effect on ensuring that C-sections are not performed for personal, professional, or institutional gain instead of clinical necessity. Beyond the obvious concern that scheduling might supersede clinical judgment, scheduled C-sections also tend to be as many as three weeks earlier than the standard forty-week pregnancy. Early delivery, of course, also comes with potentially negative consequences. In light of this, medical necessity decision making must be analyzed alongside the steadily decreasing gestational age at birth in the United States, as noted by scholars.[23] The language of a woman being "overdue" is of consequence and is a declaration that often seems to be more of a function—again—of social power's ability to establish perceived norms regarding the setting of expectations, instead of some notion of pure, evidence-based clinical judgment.[24]

The possibility of financial incentives skewing medical necessity decision making is hardly limited to the role played by physicians or other clinicians. Payers also play a role. Against the assumption that C-sections are more expensive than nonsurgical deliveries,[25] one study found the average charges for vaginal deliveries to be higher than those for C-sections.[26] Though payers may see financial incentives in the choice, a broader consideration of hospital resources—surgical resources, including operating room time, beds and amenities required during the stay—must be part of the calculus. Gruber and Owings note, "In terms of just the time investment, cesarean delivery is much more efficient for the ob-gyn; unlike normal childbirth, cesarean deliveries can be scheduled in advance, and they often take less time than a normal childbirth with extended labor."[27]

Financial dimensions are also intensified and skewed by potential litigation. Some scholars argue, for example, that C-section reduces physician liability compared to the risks of vaginal delivery.[28] There is evidence that this may be true. This argument is most clear in the case of vaginal birth after C-section (VBAC), which demonstrates the difficulty of returning to vaginal birth after a woman has delivered via C-section. The problem is that many physicians have come to believe that once women have had a C-section, returning to vaginal delivery is unduly risky because of problems with placental location and bleeding from C-section scar tissue. Theresa Morris reports that among a representative sample of women, 37 percent who have undergone a C-section had done so in a previous delivery.[29] In past years, multiple reports have indicated that insurance companies advise physicians against—and in some cases prohibit—performing VBACs. Efforts by critics of the overuse of C-sections are therefore focused on promoting vaginal deliveries for first-time mothers, which in turn reduces the perceived medical necessity of subsequent births by C-section. In arguing against VBACs, providers sometimes point to the increased resources that VBACs require.[30] This suggests that the trend against health insurance provision for VBACs may be rooted in cost calculations, and not medical judgment.

Beyond the role that physicians and payers may play, however, others argue that patients are the main driving force in high C-section rates, suggesting a perception of medical necessity among patients themselves. For example, drawing on a rhetoric of choice instead of necessity, media reports have claimed that women sometimes seek C-sections to accommodate work schedules, family travel, and other nonmedical needs.[31] Here, the ability to schedule C-sections might mark a difference between convenience and medical need, but also introduces the interpretive question of how to distinguish between them. While some physicians report that women request C-sections for nonmedical reasons, a concern also raised by an NIH study,[32] another study found that women rarely request C-sections without a significant belief in the medical necessity of the operation. This suggests that women may internalize norms from external forces and the perceived importance of medical necessity in their requests for C-sections.[33] Accordingly, the authors of one study worry that "the focus on women's request for cesarean section may divert attention away from physician-led influences on the continuing high cesarean section rates."[34] Beliefs about C-section and medical necessity—correct or incorrect—nonetheless drive patients' views. Indeed, Morris notes that 90 percent of the women represented in the study she examined reported that their C-sections were recommended by their providers for medical reasons, or at least that these women believed medical reasons to be the basis of physician recommendations.[35] This reminds us that patients are often in a quandary wherein they must on some level defer to clinicians insofar as they lack the technical training and knowledge to participate fully in clinical decision making, but are also relatively helpless to ask critical questions, resist physician advice, or seek additional perspectives when they are in the high-pressure situation of a delivery. The Morris and Wolf studies, which are two of the more recent and thorough studies available, both confirm the pervasiveness of this patient experience.

Technology also plays an important role in persuading various entities of C-section's medical necessity. For example, common views that women hold about technology and the medicalization of childbirth—namely that they are net goods—correlate closely with class indicators, as poor women trade control over childbirth, including securing the newest technologies, for access to services at the supposedly best health care facilities.[36] Access to technology becomes, in these scenarios, evidence of status, but also a source of hope that one is receiving the best care possible in the best facility.

The increased technologization of pregnancy has led to a sharp uptick in C-sections as these technologies create concerns about fetal distress. Ultrasounds in the last month of pregnancy, for example, have been found to increase the likelihood of C-section by 44 percent, and 85 percent for women whose fetuses are predicted to be—but may not actually be—large (i.e., over 7 pounds, 11 ounces).[37] Ultrasound indications in tandem with predicted weight can be problematic because they generate fears about the possibility of shoulder dystocia, a serious but rare condition that can result in permanent injury. Yet concerns that one is poised to deliver a "big baby," wrong as these predictions often are given the limitations of ultrasound for determining weight,[38] dramatically increase the chances of a C-section being declared medically necessary, even though in hindsight this determination may be revealed to be incorrect. Similarly, as Morris explains, while "nonmedically indicated inductions are commonly referred to as 'social inductions,'"[39] inductions based on predictions of presenting with a "big baby" often lead to inductions that some women realize afterwards "may not have been necessary."[40]

Perhaps the most important manifestation of the role that technology plays within medical necessity's politics of persuasion concerns electronic fetal monitoring (EFM). Though the intermittent use of EFM has provided clear benefits since its introduction in the 1970s, scholars have shown that the rise of continuous EFM—that is, EFM administered for the duration of labor—has heightened attention to perceived "fetal distress" in ways that may increase the likelihood of C-sections being deemed necessary.[41] Alarmingly, EFM is reported to yield an unacceptably high false positive rate for indications of fetal distress, to the tune of 99.8 percent.[42] The result of the use of continuous EFM has been to dramatically increase the number of C-sections without directly addressing actual cases of fetal distress. As Morris puts it, "Monitors are used to reduce legal risk, not to improve birth outcomes; yet they have been shown to unquestionably increase the c-section rate."[43]

Continuous EFM demonstrates most clearly the tensions between problems stemming from the fear of malpractice wherein EFM provides evidence that can be used against physicians in the event of health problems with newborns, and the limitations of what EFM can actually tell us. Many physicians are concerned—legitimately so, in many cases—that they will be accused of malpractice if complications arise, even if their actions had nothing to do with outcomes, especially given that fetal monitoring can be used against them in court. In her study, for example, Wolf reports multiple situations in which women were directed toward C-sections less as a result of clear instances of "fetal distress" than distress on the part of physicians.[44] This makes sense considering what we know about the politics of medical necessity. Meanwhile, other well-known and effective tools for delivery—forceps and vacuums, especially—are rarely used in large part out of concern for perceived, though often not real, complications. In addition, these trends have led to a historical agglomeration and self-fulfilling prophecy, as some years of defaulting to C-sections have eroded the knowledge base of alternative techniques, with ripple effects in medical education and during residency. The result is an increasing void of trained practitioners who have either the will or technical know-how to deliver babies vaginally.

An additional consequence of the politics of medical necessity has been an emphasis on concerns for babies' over mothers' health. As Morris puts it,

> It seems easier and less risky *to the provider* to provide a c-section. The question that should be asked is whether a c-section is easier and less risky *for the woman* than a forceps or vacuum delivery. Instead, c-sections are performed because maternity providers believe they are better protected from blame in the case of a bad outcome.[45]

This distinction of benefits accruing to providers instead of benefits accruing to women is worth meditating on. While continuous EFM and some of the other norms I have discussed are important parts of the broader politics of medical necessity that drive high C-section rates, we should not simply assess the binary of medically necessary or unnecessary. Just as important is the question of medically necessary for whom? Within the medicalized orbit of childbirth, after all, there are, at least at the point of delivery, two patients—delivering women and their babies.

The rhetoric of medical necessity that surrounds C-section is almost entirely concerned with fetal and neonatal health. In spite of this focus, C-sections have consequences for babies that suggest that litigation avoidance trumps health concerns more generally. What is clear is that the current malpractice environment, or at least institutional reactions to a perceived malpractice environment, rarely lead to the construction of a rhetoric of medical necessity that accommodates the needs of mothers as well as babies. For some mothers, of course, this trade-off may be acceptable, given the strong tendency for—and socially policed norm of—selflessness in childbirth and childrearing. But the complement of medical science and available techniques, on the one hand, and fidelity to the needs of patients, on the other, has not, within the context of C-section in

America, led to a balanced approach. Concerns about medical necessity have tended to apply mainly to fetuses and babies rather than mothers, thus the question: medical necessity for whom?

Concerned about high C-section rates, a lack of patient choice, negative long-term consequences for women, and costs, some groups have begun to take on the overuse of C-sections. The diversity of groups involved in these efforts, which includes the Centers for Disease Control and Prevention, March of Dimes, and the American College of Obstetricians and Gynecologists, signals the widespread interest in reducing the C-section rate. In some cases, such as the Centers for Disease Control and Prevention program, funding is available for hospitals engaged in efforts to reduce C-section rates. Many hospitals appear focused primarily on reducing the costs associated with medically unnecessary C-sections. In California, for example, a pilot project undertaken in three hospitals in Southern California, led by a nonprofit health business group representing public and private employers (including Disney), is seeking to reduce C-section rates. In the case of this group, which represents business, a major motivation is reducing costs associated with what they believe to be unnecessary medical care.[46] Writing in *The Atlantic* in 2015, health care reporter Anna Gorman reported on one California hospital that reduced its C-section rate from 38 percent in 2012 to 33 percent in 2015, with the number falling to 25 percent for low-risk births. They did this, moreover, simply by retraining physicians and setting new reporting and scheduling protocols. Nurses were also encouraged to work with women in labor to take measures that might reduce the likelihood of C-section, even receiving bonuses if the hospital lowered its rates to certain benchmarks. A 24-7 "laborist" program provided constant support for women in labor, especially those hoping for VBAC, which, Gorman reports, helped persuade some physicians to return to doing VBACs because the physician laborists could provide continuous support and monitoring that assuaged many of their concerns.[47]

Medical necessity and C-section is often discussed with reference to the World Health Organization's oft-cited acceptable limit point of 10 to 15 percent, above which women risk unnecessary complications, infections, lifelong consequences, and even death.[48] Medical associations, as well as the federal government, are actively seeking to reduce C-section rates through public awareness campaigns about the increased risk for complications. The NIH, for example, has called for the creation of a comprehensive website to provide information about C-section.[49] Presumably, reaching consensus about the appropriate conditions under which C-sections are warranted would mitigate some of this suspicion, though we should not be so quick to assume—as we have seen throughout this book—that the establishment of criteria would (or should) address medical necessity's challenges.

Medical necessity decision making is a function of multiple variables that are complicated and intensified by roles played by physicians, patients, and other actors.[50] While working with physicians and other clinicians involved in most American deliveries is key, the case of C-section reminds us that medical necessity requires reworking norms on the institutional level, as well as incentivizing various actors within institutions to rethink what they do and—critically for medical necessity—the rationale for why they do it. If it is the case, as Morris argues, that "the organization of the medical profession has constrained women's choices,"[51] then a reorganization of that profession must be part of the puzzle. Indeed, a goal within the politics of medical necessity is not only mindfulness about the variability and shades of gray that often accompany medical necessity decision making, but the fact that how we construct medical necessity itself has grave consequences for patients, whether they are newborn babies or pregnant or delivering mothers. The goal is therefore not only to clear away rhetorical, cultural, or institutional brush to be able to see "real" medical necessity, but to ensure that the new, more narrow conception of medical necessity becomes actualized within institutions.

Abortion: A Medical or Political Question?

American abortion politics plays out on a somewhat different (though rhetorically related) terrain than C-section.[52] However, while the medical necessity of C-section is debated by childbirth experts, the rhetoric of medical necessity arises in American abortion debates as a strategic tool, a discourse called upon not only to secure individual abortions, but to protect broader abortion rights. While norms and social power, mainly within medical institutions, play the key role in shaping C-section rates, legal rhetoric and court decisions are a—if not *the*—driving force in abortion debates.

Specifically, for reasons that concern the nature of medical necessity arguments themselves, advocates of access to safe and legal abortions often find the discourse of medical necessity useful for neutralizing contentious political dynamics. The medical frame, as we have seen in other cases, serves as a less-contentious rhetorical warrant designed to defuse or mitigate the agonistic nature of American abortion politics itself. At the same time, this creates a tension between abortion's political and medical valences. The result is that as antiabortion activists have transitioned from a scattered movement in the early twentieth century to an organized political interest in the early twenty-first,[53] American abortion politics has tended to gravitate toward medical rather than political rhetorical grounds. Accordingly, abortion rights advocates have often become mired in interpretative debates over medical necessity instead of abortion's political value. For this reason, contemporary abortion politics reveals something important about the politics of medical necessity generally.

Considering the controversy and rancor abortion elicits, we can understand the attractiveness of turning to necessity arguments. As I have explained, medical necessity's rhetorical force issues from its promise that decisions and states of being, no matter how they were arrived at, are not choices, thereby absolving individuals of responsibility for their needs and attempting to sidestep politics. This general exculpation applies as well to physicians and payers for their decision making. At the same time, this apparent stability provides a framework for shaping forms of medical knowledge that are deployable by political actors in medical debates, including physicians, patients, payers, and various actors within political movements, such as those lead by pro-choice and antiabortion groups. Consider, for example, the following statement from a prominent Canadian antiabortion group:

> Abortion is not an essential medical service. It is designated
> "medically necessary" for purely social and political, not medical,
> reasons. Pregnancy is not an "injury, illness or disease." There is no
> proof that abortion improves health. There is no "medical neces-
> sity" where no medical benefit or health risk exists.[54]

This position draws on several interrelated discourses to reject the idea that abortion is or can be medically necessary. It is worth highlighting the statement's reminder that medical necessity is a "designation," a term that evokes conscious choice as well as its grounding as a rhetorical tool.

Feminist philosopher Laura Purdy has noted, "The prochoice movement has tended to emphasize [abortion's] importance for women's health," which she regards as an understandable but "mistaken strategy."[55]

To be sure, this turn was not the product of a strategic plan by pro-choice feminists, but was foisted upon them by judicial and legislative developments that created political contexts to which they were forced to react. The emphasis on medical necessity appears to have been less of an intentional strategy than a response to judicial and legislative developments that eclipsed and obscured other forms of pro-choice argument. A brief review of these developments sheds light on a more than thirty-year reframing of the abortion question in terms of medical necessity. As with medical marijuana, many of the most prominent debates arose in a legal theater, adding a dimension of legal rhetoric and decision making to existing political and medical arguments.

The well-known 1973 decision in *Roe v. Wade* serves as the critical beginning point for understanding how medical necessity became central to American abortion politics. Though a number of frames vied for attention in the early 1970s, *Roe*, and the Texas statute it addressed, had the effect of focusing the abortion question on medical necessity, to the exclusion of other frameworks.[56] Specifically, *Roe*'s schema prohibited state regulation of first trimester abortions, allowed for some state regulation, especially for reasons of health, in the second, and allowed states to ban abortion altogether in the third, as long as such bans held exceptions for pregnant women's health. Due to the respect afforded medical judgment, under *Roe*, medical necessity, along with rape and incest exceptions, serves as the only reliable means by which abortions can be accessed during the second and third trimesters.

Scholars have noted that *Roe* "makes the physician the final arbiter of the abortion decision" beyond the first trimester.[57] Put somewhat differently, for most of a pregnancy's duration, *Roe* privileged the rights of medical professionals over those of their patients, and established principles secured by a medical framework. As the opinion holds, "subsequent to viability, the State in promoting its interest in the potentiality of human life may, if it chooses, regulate, and even proscribe, abortion except where it is necessary, in appropriate medical judgment, for the preservation of the life or health of the mother."[58] The constraining nature of *Roe*'s medical exceptions are marked precisely by the presence and prevalence of the rhetoric of necessity itself. *Roe*'s turn to medical authority was intended to neutralize the more hotly contested dimensions of pro-life and pro-choice politics, themselves important and not uncomplicated rhetorical framings. Accordingly, the turn toward the politics of medical necessity was not only pragmatic, but was a strategic effort to carve out exemptions instead of establishing politically-grounded rights. Even the decision's privacy arguments were placed under the medical umbrella, securing physician–patient relations instead of women's choice or bodily autonomy.

The focus on medical necessity was not only a product of *Roe*, but reflected arguments some pro-choice advocates made in their efforts to influence the decision. For example, a brief filed by a group of medical professionals argued,

> The Texas anti-abortion statute is wrong in principle, fundamentally unsound in the light of present day medical and surgical knowledge, and a serious obstacle to good medical practice. Amici believe that the restrictions imposed by the Texas statute on the performance of medically indicated therapeutic abortions interfere with the physician-patient relationship and with the ability of physicians to practice medicine in accordance with the highest professional standards.[59]

The brief quotes an American Psychiatric Association statement maintaining that, "A decision to perform an abortion should be regarded as strictly a medical decision and a medical responsibility." Somewhat paradoxically, however, the brief asserts that "the freedom to be the master of her own body, and thus of her own fate, is as fundamental a right as a woman can possess," thereby branding the Texas ban "the most severe and extreme invasion of her right to privacy."[60] But this turn appears as an afterthought, its ultimate appeal to privacy framed in terms of physician consultation instead of bodily autonomy.

With this medical focus firmly established, *Doe v. Bolton*, also decided in 1973, clarified how medical necessity is to be determined. Specifically, an abortion's medical necessity is a "professional judgment" that may take into consideration many "factors—physical, emotional, psychological, familial, and the women's age—relevant to the well being of the patient." The court clarified that, "All these factors may relate to health," which "allows the attending physician the room he needs to make his best medical judgment."[61] As with *Roe*, *Doe* makes physicians the arbiters of the medical necessity that govern abortion access, albeit within a fairly expansive definition of health. Yet, while both cases assert that privacy rights guarantee a woman's right to first trimester abortions, neither advances a strong political argument capable of moving beyond the confines of medicine.

The so-called Hyde Amendment of 1976, attached to the yearly congressional appropriations bill, reiterated these distinctions by prohibiting the use of federal funds to pay for "elective" abortion services, thereby reaffirming the centrality of the medical necessity question to American abortion politics. In 1977, motivated by the Hyde distinction between a woman's right to have an abortion without state intervention in the first trimester and the funding required to operationalize that right, the question of whether medical necessity determinations were enough to secure federal funding moved front and center. In these debates, questions of "state interest" and "undue burden" were largely mediated by necessity arguments, owing to a free market ideology that does not consider the inability to pay for services to constitute a substantive limitation. Hyde marks a clear decline in arguments rooted in choice.

Yet, Hyde was merely the opening move in a series of efforts to bar publicly funded abortions. In *Maher v. Roe* (1977), two women were unable to obtain a "certificate of medical necessity" required by a Connecticut welfare regulation.[62] The court found that Connecticut's unwillingness to pay for abortion services did not violate the rights established by *Roe*. The court also concluded that "it is not unreasonable for a State to insist upon a prior showing of medical necessity to insure that its money is being spent only for authorized purposes," adding that "Although similar requirements are not imposed for other medical procedures, such procedures do not involve the termination of a potential human life." In short, *Maher* found that the inability to pay for an abortion did not constitute "undue burden" and that abortion can be deemed both medically necessary and a special case that allows the state to refuse to fund it. Medical necessity declarations had been delinked from the material resources required to actualize services.[63]

Harris v. McRae (1980) marked an intensification of the rhetoric of necessity in abortion, holding that states can treat abortion as a medical procedure with unique state interest. This negated many of the benefits of the medicalized defense of abortion. Newly armed with *McRae*, the 1981 version of the Hyde Amendment decreed, "None of the funds appropriated under this Act shall be used to perform abortions except where the life of the mother would be endangered if the fetus were carried to term."[64] With this move, federal legislation intersecting with abortion was essentially reduced to medical necessity.

It is important to note the definitional games at work in Hyde renderings of medical necessity. Specifically, the various manifestations from 1976 to 1981 define medical necessity in terms of a woman's *physical* survival. It is thus insufficient to note merely that abortions not deemed medically necessary receive no federal support after *McRae*. The development of the Hyde language, which has played an important role of the narrowing of medical necessity's scope in abortion debates, includes an attempt to restrict medical necessity to physical survival but goes further to include only those conditions that "place the woman in danger of death." This turn not to life, but something closer to "bare life," evacuates medical necessity of its normative and biomedical content, replacing physicians' judgments with a "right to life."[65]

In response, several cases have tested the bounds of medical necessity exceptions to state restrictions, illustrating the inherent vulnerability and limited rhetorical utility of medical necessity as a guarantor of abortion access. In *Planned Parenthood of Southeastern Pa. v. Casey* (1992), the Supreme Court reaffirmed *Roe*'s requirement that state restrictions on postviability abortions must contain an exception, "where it is necessary, in appropriate medical judgment, for the preservation of the life or health of the mother."[66] Conjuring the politics of the archive I examined in chapter 2, *Casey* affirmed the constitutionality of record-keeping requirements, including those that could be used to question medical necessity determinations. In so doing, *Casey* intensified the possibility of postprocedure prosecution based on a reassessment of records tasked with documenting that abortion's necessity.

Casey also set the stage for a series of twenty-first-century cases that further engaged the medical necessity question. In *Stenberg v. Carhart* (2000), the court considered the constitutionality of a Nebraska statute that criminalized a rare late-term abortion procedure known as dilation and extraction (D&X). According to the statute, a D&X could not be performed "unless such procedure is necessary to save the life of the mother whose life is endangered by a physical disorder, physical illness, or physical injury, including a life-endangering physical condition caused by or arising from the pregnancy itself." To justify this lack of exception, Nebraska challenged the meaning of "necessary":

The word "necessary" in *Casey*'s phrase "necessary, in appropriate medical judgment, for the . . . health of the mother" . . . cannot refer to absolute proof or require unanimity of medical opinion. Doctors often differ in their estimation of comparative health risks and appropriate treatment. And *Casey*'s words "appropriate medical judgment" must embody the judicial need to tolerate responsible differences of medical opinion. For another thing, the division of medical opinion signals uncertainty. If those who believe that D&X is a safer abortion method in certain circumstances turn out to be right, the absence of a health exception will place women at an unnecessary risk. If they are wrong, the exception will simply turn out to have been unnecessary.[67]

Nebraska's claims underscore the extent to which debates about necessity are capable of destabilizing pro-choice positions when absolute criteria are applied to inherently contingent questions. Reproductive needs, after all, are context-bound and interpretable. More significantly, where there has been open disagreement over basic medical terms, resolutions have tended to lean toward restriction. We have seen this dynamic before, which serves as a reminder that an emphasis on necessity tends to limit rather than extend the scope of possibility and access. It is, in other words, a rhetoric that serves primarily to limit.

The case that upheld the so-called Partial-Birth Abortion Ban Act of 2003, *Gonzales v. Carhart* (known as *Carhart II*), raised similar questions and intensified the stakes of medical necessity's role within abortion politics. In contrast to *Casey*'s question of how to define medical necessity, *Carhart II* asked "whether the barred procedure is *ever* necessary to preserve a woman's health"[68] (emphasis mine) and, if not, whether the federal government had the right to ban the procedure. A *New England Journal of Medicine* editorial noted that *Carhart II* marked "the first time the Court has ever held that physicians can be prohibited from using a medical procedure deemed necessary by the physician to benefit the patient's health."[69]

Instead of reviewing the many debates contained in *Carhart II*, I focus here on the questions it raises about physicians' abilities to prove what they did and did not do and why. The following excerpt from the majority opinion is worth quoting at length. (The court uses the term D&E rather than the more familiar, colloquial D&X.)

The contention that any D&E [Dilation and Extraction] may
result in the delivery of a living fetus beyond the Act's anatomical
landmarks because doctors cannot predict the amount the cervix
will dilate before the procedure does not take account of the Act's
intent requirements, which preclude liability for an accidental intact D&E. The evidence supports the legislative determination that
an intact delivery is almost always a conscious choice rather than
a happenstance, belying any claim that a standard D&E cannot be
performed without intending or foreseeing an intact D&E. That
many doctors begin every D&E with the objective of removing
the fetus as intact as possible based on their belief that this is safer
does not prove, as respondents suggest, that every D&E might violate the Act, thereby imposing an undue burden. It demonstrates
only that those doctors must adjust their conduct to the law by not
attempting to deliver the fetus to an anatomical landmark. Respondents have not shown that requiring doctors to intend dismem-
berment before such a delivery will prohibit the vast majority of
D&E abortions.[70]

Particularly noteworthy as a corollary to the court's lack of concern with
wrongful prosecution is that it circumvents the historically and philosophically problematic question of establishing intent.[71] Again underscoring
the critical role played by the archive, *Carhart II* assumes that what physicians did or did not do can be documented in such a way that will protect
physicians from prosecution. This requires a high degree of thoroughness
in the medical record (which the Partial-Birth Abortion Ban Act treats as
evidence), including the ability to definitively ascertain whether an intact
D&X was "accidental" or "intentional."

In *Carhart II*, the majority did not take seriously the possibility that
mistakes could be read as intentional, and that intent could be read into
the normal course of a procedure considering that certain "anatomical
landmarks" may differ by fractions of inches, but fractions that mark the
difference between a lawful and unlawful action. The medical necessity of
a procedure, in other words, is bound up with the possibility of engaging
in unnecessary—and under *Carhart II* unlawful—activity.[72] The question
of intent becomes a matter not of medical judgment or Hippocratic fidelity, but a retrospective legal determination. Though determining what

happened is the foundation of *Carhart II*'s prosecutorial charge, the opinion makes clear that "what happened" is no simple matter.

These cases set the stage for more recent developments that arose within the context of Obama-era health care reform. In the summer of 2009, the Obama administration's efforts had become mired in controversy over whether federal funds would be used to pay for abortions. A group of conservative legislators organized by Democratic representative Bart Stupak made its support for health care reform contingent on the inclusion of the following language:

> No funds authorized or appropriated by the Act (or amendment made by this Act) may be used to pay for any abortion or to cover any part of the costs of any health plan that includes coverage of abortion, except in the case where a woman suffers from a physical disorder, physical injury, or physical illness that would, as certified by a physician, place the woman in danger of death unless an abortion is performed, including a life-endangering physical condition caused by or arising from the pregnancy itself, or unless the pregnancy is the result of an act of rape or incest.[73]

Though it was not ultimately included in the final version of the ACA, Stupak's language (which came to be known as the Stupak-Pitts amendment) marks the rhetorical position that antiabortion is an ultimate horizon within the politics of medical necessity. Ultimately, President Obama won passage of the ACA by bargaining with Stupak and issuing an executive order upon passage of the bill that provided an "adequate enforcement mechanism to ensure that federal funds are not used for abortion services (except in cases of rape or incest, or when the life of the woman would be endangered), consistent with a longstanding federal statutory restriction that is commonly known as the Hyde Amendment."[74] In other words, President Obama's assurances merely restated the Hyde language to satisfy a political need while essentially maintaining the status quo in policy terms.

The developments I have described illustrate the risks associated with reducing abortion rights to medical necessity arguments. Petchesky identified the problem some years ago, noting that "Medical necessity . . . may be used to expand women's access to necessary reproductive health services or to restrict women's sphere of action in favor of parents' or physicians' authority."[75] To be sure, *Roe*'s medical necessity framework has *mostly* held. Yet, the political force of this holding has been largely gutted by efforts to redefine necessity.[76] Post-*Roe* necessity arguments have become synonymous with women's survival to the exclusion of more holistic and contemporary conceptions of health. They certainly do not value wellness or preventive health services. This development makes clear that medical necessity arguments cannot be assumed to carry with them the force that earlier abortion rights advocates assumed they would. The lesson concerns the limits of the medical necessity frame in abortion and other contentious political domains. This lesson, as well, underscores the costs of evoking medical necessity as well as the potential of leaning on the rhetoric of medical necessity as part of a political strategy.

Though C-section and abortion raise different questions about medical necessity, taken together they provide an opportunity to deepen our understanding of the intersections of gender, reproduction, and the politics of medical necessity. I offer this analysis in the spirit of the rhetorical tradition's conviction that thinking through phenomena that are sometimes quite different, but share rhetorical structures, patterns, or themes, can bear analytic fruit.[77]

It is therefore worth noting a few shared dynamics. First, critics of C-section and abortion both seek a decline in their frequency, which in turn encourages a critical rethinking of medical necessity. In both cases, medical necessity is used as a limiting concept, even as pro-choice advocates hope that medical necessity will be able to hold a line in protecting abortion rights. Critics of both, as well, raise questions about how medical necessity is defined and justified. Conversely, it is worth noting that few participants in these debates actively advocate an increase in either procedure. Indeed, rates of both abortion and C-section appear to be declining.[78] While there is a clear reason for the decline in the former, which is largely attributed to increased access to birth control, especially through the ACA, declining C-section rates are both less dramatic and surrounded by less certainty regarding causality. Nonetheless, it is worth taking note of the trajectories of both as they are clearly bound up in the rhetoric of medical necessity.

There are, of course, major differences between C-section and abortion as regards their orientation toward reproduction. The former aims to see a pregnancy through to birth while the latter is concerned with termination.

They are, to this extent, lodged in quite different political and moral discourses, and are laden with different meanings. The role that medical interventions play, guided by the rhetoric of medical necessity, is therefore distinct. For example, though abortion is regarded by many pro-choice advocates as a cornerstone of women's health, the role that physicians play in carrying out abortions is often treated in a quite different way than C-section. While there is a burgeoning movement to work with physicians to lower C-section rates, scholars also tend to regard unnecessary C-sections as a systemic problem encouraged by forces far greater than physician or patient choices. This is consistent, of course, with my focus on power/knowledge throughout this book. The manifestations of these forces include the role of medical malpractice laws and patient perceptions of benefits of C-section, institutional norms regarding the use of fetal monitoring, the consequences of team-based care and consultation with maternal-fetal high-risk pregnancy specialists, whose very consultation can be used in court as evidence of a problem.

One key difference must be punctuated in the clearest possible terms. Though the negative consequences of high C-section rates are real, and the passions of critics of high C-section rates run high, I do not know of any instances in which a physician was threatened for performing one, as numerous physicians who perform abortions have been and continue to be.[79] Indeed, physicians, most notably Dr. George Tiller in 2009,[80] have been killed for performing what they regard as an important service for women's health. The stakes of the politics of medical necessity in these two areas of reproductive politics are quite different, even though both are of real consequence for women's health.

More generally, there is also a key difference between the politics of medical necessity and C-section in that some antiabortion opponents, at a limit point, aim to prove that abortion is never medically necessary— even in the historically acknowledged exceptions of rape, incest, and in situations where the pregnant woman's life is believed to be in danger— while the most vocal critic of C-sections would never maintain such a position. Indeed, while medical necessity exceptions that license abortion are being actively targeted by antiabortion advocates, critics of skyrocketing C-section rates acknowledge several areas where C-section is clearly medically necessary, as in the case of placenta previa (when a placenta covers the cervix), or when women have cardiac conditions that make pushing dangerous.[81] What critics of unnecessary C-sections want above all is to make vaginal birth the default, and to take active measures to increase the likelihood of vaginal delivery. They seek, for example, to challenge the routine use of continuous EFM, to seek reforms in malpractice law as well as institutional cultures, and to demedicalize childbirth to the greatest extent possible, which would in turn return C-section to what they regard as its proper place as a relatively rare medical intervention in only the most serious cases.

The lessons for understanding the rhetoric of medical necessity are instructive. Though advocates of safe and accessible abortion have in recent decades turned to medical necessity arguments as an attempt to prevent further erosion of *Roe*-era protections, medical necessity itself is a stopgap measure. The rhetorical appeal to medical necessity is intended as a means of branding antiabortion advocates as endangering women's lives and making decisions about their bodies in situations when women may need an abortion. This approach, however, renders moot historically established rhetorical positions that secured access to abortions by appealing to the liberal notions of rights and choices. In addition, as medical technology advances and new life-saving measures are introduced into the medical repertoire, it is possible that a politics of abortion based largely on medical necessity will undermine completely the argument for maintaining patient–physician decision making about abortion. In the case of abortion, we see clearly the effects of exchanging political argumentation— especially that of the framework of rights and choice—for the rhetoric of medical necessity.

Unlike abortion, the politics of C-section is driven by a desire by critics to see clarity in medical necessity itself. Medical necessity is, in a sense, the central front in C-section debates which, compared with abortion, seems appropriate. There is, moreover, in C-section debates something of a more principled concern with medical necessity than abortion debates allow. It is not clear, in other words, that many actors within C-section debates are a priori concerned with proving the medical necessity of C-section; rather, C-section medical necessity debates are riddled by misinformation, litigious forces (some real, others perceived), and institutional and group decision-making dynamics. The forces I have described—concerns about malpractice, the uses of technology, and questions about convenience, among others—have all made it difficult to see what we might call "real" or "actual" medical necessity. By returning to basics, and rethinking the identifying features and appropriate conditions of medically necessary

C-sections themselves, these critics seem to think C-section rates will fall and medical necessity will return to its proper medical and rhetorical position as a procedure of last resort, and only in carefully delineated, evidence-based situations.

As I noted at the outset, the intersections of sexuality, gender, and reproduction are fairly predictable sites of contention within American medical necessity debates. While they might be predictable, however, excluding an analysis of them from a book on the politics of medical necessity would be odd. These issues are, after all, some of the most contentious sites of debate, and therefore an important piece of how medical necessity commonly appears in American medical debates concerned with reproduction. What I have attempted to do here is less to review the issues from the beginning, comprehensively or exhaustively, than to emphasize some of the ways in which each reveals unique dynamics of medical necessity discourse.

Conclusion

Embracing the Politics of Medical Necessity

This book seeks to answer three fundamental questions. First, why is the rhetoric of medical necessity so central to American medicine, and how did it come to be so? Second, what strategies have been called upon to interpret medical necessity, and to what effect? Third, what are the political, social, economic, legal, and other implications of the discourse's prevalence, and in what direction do these implications point us as we consider how to approach medical necessity in future debates? From the vantage point I have sought to establish, medical necessity appears to be a quite different phenomenon than that acknowledged by the vast majority of scholars who have studied it. My analysis points to a need for jettisoning longstanding attempts to define medical necessity, or focusing only on formal processes and procedures, and instead engaging a politics of medical necessity in a more transparent fashion. Such a politics would allow for a social response in which the various stakeholders—from clinicians to patients, industries to elected officials, ethicists to policy analysts—negotiate the boundaries of medical priorities as the United States attempts to develop a more effective health care system.

In a sense, my key contribution is likely to be an epistemic shift. Simply seeing medical necessity for what it is and approaching it with clarity is an important step that could in and of itself yield dividends. As I have argued, the more people gain access to health care services, the more the stakes of medical necessity debates rise. Assuming we reach, perhaps at some distant point, universal coverage in the United States, only a more thoughtful approach to medical necessity, construed broadly, can ensure a sustainable, ethical, and effective system.

The more recent politics to which the ACA has given rise shines a light on coverage gaps that exclude millions of Americans from making medical necessity claims in the first place. If the United States moves toward universality, be it through a national health care system on the order of a single-payer or "Medicare for All" program or simply a more comprehensive patchwork than currently exists, this could afford individuals a voice in thinking about how these actors understand the technical terms with which they are confronted by health care institutions. It is important, from the perspective of civic participation, that key stakeholders think about necessity in general, and medical necessity in particular, within a context that includes their needs as well as the needs of others. This is especially important if scarce resources are presumed. If they are not presumed, a rethinking of the resourcing of medical needs is in order. Even so, as no approach is purely objective, every theory of medical necessity will need to wrestle with the degree of subjectivity it wishes to allow in determining the appropriateness of social supports for medical services.

There are major unknowns: for example, what dynamics— technological, economic, social, and beyond—will characterize medical necessity's future? And how will stakeholders within the medical establishment respond to the contention that medicine is, at base, political? It is critical to remember that all health care systems use medical necessity in various ways and to different degrees. This fact suggests that mere dependence on certain conceptual tools does not determine the nature of that concept's rhetorical deployments.

It follows that the rhetoric of medical necessity is always embedded in and shaped by political contexts. American political culture embraces the rhetorics of individuality and personal responsibility, which have important consequences for medical necessity. Within this political culture, claims made by individuals from certain groups—usually members of racial and sexual minorities, but also women and the disabled—are cast in specifically suspicious lights that give their medical necessity claims less traction. Such people are differently placed precisely because they must evoke medical arguments to secure basic health care services, whether they are unique to them or not.

The future of medical necessity depends in large part on the development of the interpretive culture appended to it, where interpretation takes place as a contest arising within and in tension with power. Thus, while "the medical" and "necessity" may suggest certain intuitive entailments, such as that all emergencies constitute situations wherein a state of necessity is present, the more salient question is not so much what medical necessity does as what political actors do with it. Such an approach recognizes the consequences of turning to either restrictive or expansive interpretations, and makes those consequences part of the political discussion. Finally, this approach jettisons the fantasy of establishing a health care system without trade-offs. This jettisoning not only enables us to acknowledge costs and benefits, but recognizes that all perceived necessities cannot be recognized as such in a system based on fairness, equity, and universality.

Focusing on the rhetorical production of medical necessity exposes the divide between different perceptions of medical need—those of patients and physicians, for example—and the ways in which American health care institutions have turned to medical necessity to frame medical priorities and constrain the conceptual boundaries of legitimate and illegitimate care. Such a focus can also tell us a great deal about how patients, communities, physicians, insurance companies, and other actors are variously respected, trusted, and accorded powers, with wildly different levels of autonomy, to shape health care utilization. Once we are clear that the turn to medical necessity was not only pragmatic, but political, we can see why sustained political engagement with medical necessity is essential to developing a health care system that meets basic public health objectives.

Instead of merely cataloging normative positions, the view of medical necessity with which I wish to leave readers emphasizes a procedural disposition toward medical necessity—a method for approaching, analyzing, and studying it. In taking this approach, to return again to Foucault, it is important to avoid advancing or indulging in a "unitary discourse" about medical necessity that while satisfying an urge to have something concrete or fixed, would lead us further away from understanding medical necessity itself. This arms-length approach, maintained in the name of critical distance, helps us to avoid hoisting—in Foucault's terms—a "halo of theory that would unite" medical necessity's various threads above the actual, often daily, and ever-changing struggles that comprise the politics of medical necessity itself.[1] Given medical necessity's complexity as well as the dimensions of social power that underpin medicine itself, there can be no grand theory of medical necessity. The hoisting of a halo would only serve to misrepresent medical necessity as it is actually found at specific decision points. Eschewing artificial theoretical unity leaves the question of medical necessity open in order to be able to engage the particular struggles that comprise the larger whole. It is, in other words, always a work in progress. This approach allows us to let go of the fantasy of establishing far-reaching, all-encompassing theoretical frameworks that attempt to place all medical necessity decision making under one umbrella, and focus instead on the rhetorical moments, the shifting of forces, and the microlevel contestations that comprise the totality of attempts to determine medical necessity.

What, then, is the future of medical necessity? Developments such as genetics and comparative effectiveness research promise to remove some of the uncertainty that judgment introduces into clinical decision making by creating modes of care that are regarded as increasingly objective, suggesting that the days of viewing medicine as an art as well as a science may be numbered. But, as we should expect, this aspiration is primarily achieved through rhetorical strategies that operate in a misguided and inadequately theorized epistemic field. Aspirations that allow the idea of medical necessity to cohere with a more fixed, stable future are themselves products of a theoretical horizon based on problematic premises. The attainment of an objective medical necessity standard hinges on a promise. Unfortunately, medical necessity's rhetorical thrust—of fixity and objectivity—always exceeds that promise.

Casting medical necessity as a rhetorical production shows that the concept can serve as a guide for making sense of the multiple configurations and sites of power that govern American health care. Framing medical necessity in this way also shows why the rhetoric of medical necessity is insufficient for realizing contemporary health care objectives. But, since it is entrenched in American health care delivery on the specific level of determining who gets what and why, the politicization of medical necessity's definitional boundaries must become a central part of health care advocacy and agitation. This requires coming to terms with the political nature of the medical as well as the medical nature of the political. It means surrendering the dream of attaining a value-neutral means of regulating health care utilization—as health policy scholar Andrew Ward, for example, does when he advocates "focusing on value-neutral needs as opposed to subjective preferences"[2]—and directing our energies instead toward a sustained engagement with those values. This approach adjusts the focus of medical necessity debates, removing them from unnoticed rhetorical and epistemic roots so that theorists, practitioners, and policymakers alike can better understand medical necessity's political and biopolitical implications.

Nonetheless, numerous stakeholders continue to attempt to avoid this political thicket by developing conceptual frameworks that seek to regulate health care utilization while eschewing the hopelessly abstract medical necessity. We have seen that libertarian critics tend to link medical necessity's vagueness to the specter of frivolous lawsuits and moral hazard, noting, for example, that when patients sue on the basis of such vague promises they tend to win. We have seen, as well, the role that continuous electronic fetal monitoring plays in facilitating legal actions rooted in retrospectively constructed medical necessity claims. To avoid such actions, some critics turn to contracts in the hopes of minimizing the definitional murkiness often associated with medical necessity. The idea behind this approach is to provide patients with a clear sense of what is covered and what is not, thereby circumventing subjective debates. Implicit in this approach is a concession to the inevitable failure of projects intended to define medical necessity, but also a belief that definitional findings would be unlikely to be operationalized anyway, leading to wide variation in the construction of medical necessity as applied. Before turning to a discussion of what a political approach to medical necessity involves, I examine three common attempts to escape medical necessity's political dimensions.

Contracts

Medical necessity's failure to attain its rhetorical promise of objectivity has given rise to a range of policy proposals aimed at stabilizing the discourse. Some critics have proposed that contracts may be best-positioned to circumvent medical necessity's definitional politics. The idea is to move away from the hopelessly expansive question of what is or is not medically necessary to a legal arrangement in which parties·to contracts are clear on specific terms instead of an abstract notion of medical necessity. This approach requires a concession to the fact that necessity emphasizes agreement rather than fixed principles. Instead of utilizing an ambiguous concept, advocates of this approach counsel detailing which treatments are and are not to be covered under specific conditions, and making this information the basis of a marketplace in which health care consumers can purchase a package of available health services that they find suitable. This consumer-oriented approach is intended to neutralize the thorny problem of medical decision making in the face of particular treatment requests, replacing it instead with a list of available services and contexts in which they will be provided. In this approach, transparency is cast as a critical first step toward affording greater choice and patient preference in selecting plans. It is not only part of a general approach to medical necessity, but part of a consumer-based movement in American medicine.

Though this approach acknowledges the insufficiency of defining medi-cal necessity in the abstract, it maintains a degree of risk and, somewhat paradoxically in light of its aims, contingency. Its primary mechanism is shifting responsibility for risk to consumers. Morreim underscores the choices that must be made within this framework by advocating "guidelines-based contracting" that "jettison[s] the notion of medical necessity and the vague promises of providing 'all the care you need.'"[3] Specifically, he argues that medical necessity rubrics should be replaced with guidelines that "lay open to consumers the clinical guidelines by which [insurers] make benefit determinations, explain the procedures by which the guidelines will change over time, describe the procedures they use to adjudicate disputes and re-solve ambiguous cases, and then make those guidelines and procedures the explicit basis on which they contract with enrollees."[4] Despite the attrac-tiveness of the promised stability and transparency, the proposed turn to contracts also introduces new problems. Contracts—especially in a compli-cated domain such as health care—often lack effective mechanisms for ad-judicating fairness, especially on markets that are by nature asymmetrical, where insurers possess far greater understanding of insureds' likely needs than the insureds themselves.[5] The fairness to which they tend to point often depends on disclosing terms in pages upon pages of legalese—hardly a fair way to inform customers.

In interpreting these contracts and mediating disputes, the legal prin-ciple of *contra proferentem* plays an important role. *Contra proferentem* ("against the offerer") holds that situations in which ambiguous language, lacking resolution through other interpretive approaches,[6] is to be con-strued against the drafters of contracts. This principle is generally held to be one of fairness in large part because drafters possess superior power in comparison to those subject to the contracts they draft. Also at issue is the unequal position in which signatories to contracts often find them-selves, especially with regard to "contracts of adhesion" composed largely of "boilerplate terms that are proffered by sophisticated commercial enti-ties and ordinarily accepted by professional unsophisticated consumers."[7] *Contra proferentem*, according to one legal expert,

> is not intended to identify the most balanced outcome, ex post,
> nor to follow the most common market arrangement. Instead, it is
> intended to induce the drafter to make drafting choices that would

not overreach and would not necessitate court intervention in the first place.[8]

Contra proferentem poses problems for insurance companies who are likely to lose challenges to denials for services that physicians deem medically necessary for their patients, if those denials refer to medical necessity standards that are not specified with great detail. Accordingly, in early challenges to HMO medical necessity denials, *contra proferentem* often led to erring on the side of patients and their physicians' abilities to secure services that they thought were necessary, even if not explicitly contained in contractual language.[9] Yet, as is to be expected, insurers became savvy in response to courts' deference to patients and physicians, and drafted increasingly detailed and complex contracts.[10]

While the use of detailed contracts provided insurers with new tools for counterbalancing *contra proferentem*, it only further complicated the politics of medical necessity. As Gregg Bloche notes, "according trump value to people's ex ante health care choices—the decisions they make, often by default, when they buy health insurance—is at odds with core human needs that we look to medical care to meet."[11] The vagueness of medical necessity, long understood to be a conceptual framework that depends on an ethos of fairness, had increasingly become a battleground of contract drafting in which lawyers sought to plug as many holes as possible. Contracts have become longer and more difficult to understand to the layperson, constituting a clear setback from patient perspectives to the extent that they contain fewer opportunities for patients and their advocates to exploit ambiguity. They also devised strategies aimed at contracting out of *contra proferentem* by including language in which both parties disavow any disadvantage in construing the terms of the contract.

It is important to note that those who tend to advocate contracts as a way out of medical necessity's vagueness also tend to reject regulatory mechanisms necessary to ensure the fairness of contracts as concerns their ability to meet insureds' health needs. Much of the literature I have engaged above exists as part of a probusiness effort to correct what its adherents regard as an imbalance in contract law that empowers patients, physicians, and beyond against the interests of insurance companies who, in their view, conform to the basic rules of market-based insurance. It nonetheless remains the case that such an approach depends upon certain assumptions about the ability for market signals to produce actuarially sound insurance products as well as the presence of symmetrical knowledge between the insurer and insured in making mutually agreeable decisions about medical necessity. The focus on asymmetry and challenges in resolving ambiguity reminds us that contracts often obscure power relations.[12] Evidence shows that consumers do not always make better decisions about their care when they have more options on insurance markets, but are often only left confused without choosing a plan that is optimal for them.[13] On the other hand, fewer plans with more predictability as to what they cover appears to serve patients better, with less room for misunderstanding how medical necessity is deployed within them. Regardless of their explanatory comprehensiveness, contracts are not an answer to problems posed by the politics of medical necessity.

Rights

Some scholars have turned to the rhetorical appeal of rights to attempt to circumvent the politics of medical necessity. Rights would seem to succeed where contracts fail precisely because they promise outcomes. For example, feminist theorists Corrêa, Petchesky, and Parker argue that "human rights offer the most viable rhetorical structure currently available to civil society groups for making social and erotic justice claims and seeking redress or accountability."[14] If they are correct, then it is worth asking, especially considering the volatility of medical knowledge and the vulnerability of medical subjects within these systems, whether it might be worth exchanging necessity arguments for rights.

The rights-based approach is appealing for a few reasons. First, it "provides both the norms upon which movements can base social justice claims and shame corporate and government violators—even when, in practice, enforcement is weak." Second, it possesses a force that market-based approaches lack, largely "because they are ethically closed systems; that is, they measure value only by private preferences or by price, with the lowest costs having the highest value."[15] In this view, rights-based approaches can call attention to relations of power and other political dynamics in ways that other approaches cannot, implying "duties, not charity."[16] This is because, as Deborah Stone has noted, "rights work by dramatizing power relationships as personal stories, by legitimizing political demands, by mobilizing new political alliances, and, eventually, by transforming social institutions."[17] In a sense, we have seen this kind of politics arise out of the backlash to managed care, in which insurance denials were exposed in rather public forums—such as filmmaker Michael Moore's film about the U.S. health care system, *Sicko*. A rights-based approach may be capable of looking beyond, for example, injustice in insurance denials, by creating a picture of what a just health care system would look like when human rights are afforded primacy. A right is a political claim that can be defended as part of what a people value. The ability of this general approach to secure resources for those in need—where need is understood expansively and in a culturally diverse, context-dependent sense—rises and falls on its ability to persuade various parties of its importance. The standard does not therefore reduce to successful references to objective need, ability to navigate coding regimes, or relative position vis-à-vis biomedical or scientific developments. Its reference point is more expansive and socially meaningful.

This consideration of rights has something potentially important to contribute to our understanding of the politics of medical necessity. At base, concern about the volatility of needs-based arguments actually seems to stem from necessity's dependency on other forms of knowledge—available scientific information, technological sophistication, and even deservedness. In other words, medical necessity derives its force from ancillary discourses, which makes them contingent and dependent—vulnerable to epistemic shifts—and therefore always potentially unable to stand on their own. To again evoke Stone, "like all policy instruments, rights depend on larger politics for their effectiveness."[18] The paradox here is that most theorists of medical necessity turn to the concept precisely because of its purported concreteness, especially when compared to traditionally-recognized political categories such as justice. Rights, on the other hand, appear to be comparatively self-standing, sustained politically, and do not therefore depend "on the beneficence of unnamed, impersonal forces—whether they be donors, the state, an abstract 'society,' or, more tenuously still, the market."[19]

Given their well-documented history of being insufficient responses to contentious political problems, we must also acknowledge the limitations of rights-based approaches. For example, it may be the case that while certain claims may be best made in terms of rights—such as, perhaps, disability arguments—others, because of their tensions with (for example) religious beliefs in the area of sexuality or dominant gender norms, may be forced to appeal to necessity, even when these arguments are unlikely to secure the ultimate grounds advocates seek.

For example, writing on common health care needs among transgender people, Judith Butler notes, "At least in the United States where socialized medicine is largely understood as a communist plot, it won't be an option to have the state or insurance companies pay for these procedures without first establishing that there are serious and enduring medical and psychiatric reasons for doing so."[20] The medicalization that underpins medical necessity, in other words, contains the power to "mobilize social resources"[21] in specific situations. Following Casper and Clarke's approach to medicalization, which "assumes that 'rightness' and 'wrongness' are socially constructed, partial, and contingent,"[22] how we understand medical necessity bears not only on American health care, but political culture more generally, of which the muted reception of rights is an important part. In some cases, medical necessity will be capable of mobilizing wider support than rights claims. The question of whether we would prefer to regard such social resources as addressing specifically medical needs is often beside the point when the central aim is to secure important resources for those in need of care.

Though rights claims may sometimes be superior to necessity arguments for securing access to care, in entertaining the role that rights may play we must heed the Derridean warning that "rights by themselves are necessary but insufficient to meet the demands of justice."[23] No one strategy can overcome all challenges associated with securing medical care within political orders characterized by a strong faith in market forces and a formidable presence of conservatives who continually seek to slash social programs. The turn to rights has also historically introduced additional problems such as competition among groups seeking recognition and unproductive in-fighting over the resources that rights entail. Finally, there is the longstanding problem that critics of rights have noted, in that rights tend to be simultaneously supportive of some groups while excluding others. Accordingly, if rights are to be considered as an alternative (or supplement) to the politics of medical necessity, such considerations must be made strategically and in full awareness of their limitations and complications.

Technology

To many critics, technology constitutes one of the most exciting means of avoiding medical necessity's political dimensions and grounding defenses of health care utilization in objective criteria. To this extent, technology plays a role in medical necessity debates not unlike that which it plays in other domains of politics and policy, such as the "promethean" impulse that some scholars have identified in environmental politics, in which technological fixes might allow us to address climate change without altering the way in which we live.[24] In a way that mirrors a dynamic I have emphasized throughout this book, such an approach attempts—understandably—to minimize the messiness of social and political engagement while maintaining current behaviors and processes. Yet flawed thinking undermines the belief that technology can mitigate medical necessity's political challenges. This approach creates something of a feedback loop precisely because technology not only shapes what is and is not possible, it is constitutive of what ends up becoming seen as medically necessary. In other words, technology is a product of our social relations and not a simple addendum to them.[25] As technology becomes more sophisticated, many actors hope that medical necessity determinations will become increasingly specific and customized, but also more accurate. To this extent, there is great hope in some quarters that technology will mitigate at least some of the problems associated with the establishment of medical necessity criteria.

Consider the discovery of the BRCA 1 and 2 genes, which indicate the likelihood that some women will develop breast cancer. This genetic technology is making it easier to identify future cancer patients before symptoms arise. But, as with all technological developments, there is still considerable room for debate in terms of the significance of these findings, especially as regards the proper strategy for intervening before cancer's onset. At the same time as we are benefiting from the arrival of genomic sophistication, routine screenings for breast cancer for women without genetic predisposition are being rethought. Specifically, some breast cancer advocates fear that changes in routine mammography protocols are being established for purposes of cost savings instead of sound evidence-based clinical judgment—a possibility that we should by no means discount.[26] Some widely used chemotherapy regimens are also being questioned, with a call for the use of DNA in better targeting patients who will actually benefit from them.[27] Even as questions about the role that clinical as well as financial value plays in medical necessity decision making raise concerns among advocates of access to breast cancer screenings, biomedical researchers seek to establish a sustainable and effective regimen for detecting and treating breast cancer.[28] These efforts include—in a way that echoes continuous electronic fetal monitoring debates—resisting routine mammography for patients without family histories or other risk factors, in an effort to avoid unnecessary surgery resulting from false positives as well as unnecessary radiation exposure. The United States Preventive Services Task Force has clarified that the standards for routine mammography should not apply to those patients with a family history of breast cancer or other risk factors.[29] In other words, this approach to medical necessity is discursive, with quite different dimensions playing key roles in establishing the persuasive force of mammography's medical necessity or lack thereof.

Genetics promise to clarify medical necessity by tethering judgment to one's unique code. Yet, this promise raises a new question: can or should one be granted access to expensive and invasive medical services based on a predicted future need? If so, what is the basis of the persuasive force of genetics? While most of the relevant studies do not consider cost as a clinically-relevant factor (federally funded comparative effective research is forbidden from considering cost, for example) the current expense of genetic testing and preparation of genetically specific treatments, compounded by medical interventions such as preventive mastectomies, will surely find their way into the politics of medical necessity. More to the point, however, is the question of whether genetic testing quells or excites the politics of medical necessity. Specifically, does knowing more, and being more precise, help us to determine what is and is not necessary?

Technology drawing on genetic testing carries with it a range of consequences for health care financing. Moving forward, this will be an important part of the broader American health care discussion, affecting insurance provision, social dispositions toward the role of genomic testing and therapies, financing, and comparative effectiveness assessments that ultimately bear on medical necessity decision making. As Haga and Willard argue,

> Other challenges that affect the economic influence of genome technologies include lack of oversight, limited uptake due to fears of genetic discrimination, determination of medical necessity and

who should be tested, and the absence of immediate benefit. The high costs of some tests that might benefit only a small group will create a difficult dilemma for health-care and insurance administrators, given the rapidly rising health-care expenditures.[30]

Clearly, the increasing introduction of genomic research in a medical system characterized by a strong presence of economic interests poses real challenges. Antidiscrimination protections and other forms of oversight will play an important role. The more that genomic research is used to justify medical necessity decision making, the more we should expect pushback from payers. Genetic testing of course holds great promise for aiding physicians in the promotion of less aggressive but increasingly effective and more targeted care. But what is its significance to the political dimensions of medical necessity decision making? Does it stand to achieve the longstanding goal of depoliticizing medical necessity? What is the persuasive force of genetics?

Once again, with medical necessity it is important to attend closely to language. In response to concerns about overtesting for patients with prostate cancer at low risk of advancing, a Cleveland Clinic report celebrates a new genetic test to "help your doctor more accurately determine just how aggressive your cancer is—and whether surgery or radiation therapy is truly necessary."[31] The test aims to accomplish this by measuring the expression levels of seventeen genes across four biological pathways to predict the aggressiveness of a man's prostate cancer. Yet, there is reason to believe that the impact of this technology on medical necessity's political dimensions is likely to be muted. In fact, such technologies may intensify rather than temper disagreement over medical necessity, despite clear potential benefits. Specifically, attempts to temper or control the discourse of medical necessity by introducing ancillary discourses—such as genetics and genomics—add new voices that only serve to make that debate more excitable. They also introduce new costs that increase the political and economic stakes of expanding the scope of medical necessity to include them.

American medicine is unprepared to engage the questions that expanding frontiers of genetics and genomics have already begun to open. The National Institutes of Health spends more on genetic research than almost any other area[32] and the discourses of health care utilization center increasingly on genetics and genomics.[33] As medical science transforms, it will encounter the issues of particularity that medical necessity raises. This vision was articulated in the Precision Medicine Initiative launched during the Obama administration, which promised "a bold new research effort to revolutionize how we improve health and treat disease," which it proposed to do through a $215 million investment in "a new model of patient-powered research that promises to accelerate biomedical discoveries and provide clinicians with new tools, knowledge, and therapies to select which treatments will work best for which patients." In his announcement, President Obama distinguished between a "'one-size-fits-all' approach," and precision medicine's focus on accounting for "individual differences in people's genes, environments, and lifestyles."[34] The program, in its current manifestation, is exploring ways to enroll children to study genomic disposition and development across the life course.[35] It is unknown how the Trump administration will alter these Obama-era priorities.

However, with a greater personalization of medicine, the future of medical necessity must lie in the development of individualized regimens of medical necessity. And, if individualization does not become more affordable, it is likely to intensify inequality in medicine. The result will be a more fine-grained, yet comparatively inaccessible, understanding of medical necessity rather than an understanding that leads to calculable health outcomes. Advances such as precision medicine do stand to alter the politics of medical necessity, but such alterations will not depoliticize medical necessity itself.[36]

Political disagreement and the proliferation of persuasive dimensions are closely related. For example, a California health care provider was sued successfully over inappropriate denials for cancer surgeries on the basis of medical necessity. A *Los Angeles Times* article explained, "New advances in technology and surgical procedures often lead to disagreements among medical professionals over the proper course of treatment for some complex cases."[37] The reality of this increasingly technological future will be one of proliferating discourse, with the need for tarrying with new rhetorical structures.

These developments also raise new specters of abuse, open new doors for discrimination, and have the potential to give health insurance actuaries the ability to use genetic data to predict an entire life trajectory of costly health expenditures. Similar critiques about the misuse of data and its impact on privacy have been made about workplace wellness programs.[38] These examples illustrate the double-edged nature of data. This is true despite civil liberties protections, including those passed as part of the ACA, as the enforcement of existing mechanisms remains a problem. Only a fraction of violation charges made under the Health Insurance Portability and Accountability Act of 1996 (HIPAA), which controls this area of regulatory oversight, have actually resulted in investigations, and even fewer have led to prosecutions, in large part due to understaffing in the Department of Health and Human Services Office for Civil Rights. There is some indication that this is now changing, however, and enforcement is expected to increase.[39]

The focus on genetics also lends itself to the further individualization and privatization of health care utilization debates. This is a trend that has long been attributed to the neoliberalization of social goods, where social responsibility is reduced to individual responsibility. Debates need to consider the utilization of social resources—such as air and water quality—because it is important to consider the social causes of such individual needs. It is critical to consider not only genetics and genomics, but epigenetics, which underscore the extent to which genetic dispositions are functions of interactions with social conditions. Attempts to reduce the politics of medical necessity to individual choices not only fall short, but obscures the social basis of individual need itself. At stake in these debates is whether medical necessity's ability to minimize the effect of personal responsibility narratives is retained, with the effect being that medical necessity itself becomes less effective in securing health care services and equipment. Turning to technology in the hope of evading the social dimensions of the politics of medical necessity only results in illustrating those dimensions' centrality to technology, as well as technology's ability to conceal and repress the truths within other systems of power.[40]

It is not enough to argue that increased precision will afford patients greater control over decision making about their health, quality of life, or end of life. Nor is it wise to assume that increased technical capacity will ensure better outcomes through enhanced clinical and technical control. Precision must be evaluated in relation to its capacity to connect bodies on their level of particularity with the whole range of tools available to institutional power. This dynamic then creates sites for the potential repression and liberation of medical subjects. Precise analytics with more sophisticated medical necessity regimes do not resolve the problems that this book has explored.

Those who evoke medical arguments in political contests may find themselves and their causes subjected to unwanted medicalization. In the area of reproductive politics, for example, only with the onset of assisted reproductive technologies did "involuntary childlessness become medicalized."[41] Similarly, sonograms may be used to provide much needed information about the status of developing fetuses, but can also be used to manipulate women considering whether or not to have an abortion. Technical capacity to nurture a first trimester fetus to viability and term may be evoked to negate certain rights altogether.

Medical necessity is therefore not a mere question of which technologies are available and what benefits and risks they may present, but of the related political discourses with which they intersect. As technologies change, necessity arguments established in relation to outdated technologies may be deemed no longer necessary. For this reason alone, although the evocation of necessity arguments may constitute a compromise to political realities, a need to work within existing power relations, and a pragmatic tool for securing short-term gains, the ultimate goal should be to secure arguments on political grounds, beyond any fixed notion of medical necessity.

Contextualizing Evidence, Working with Norms

These misguided or insufficient attempts to evade medical necessity's normative dimensions make clear that instead of attempting to circumvent them, we must embrace and engage the normative foundations of medical necessity decision making. Many of the cases I have examined center on the negotiation of normatively infused elective, cosmetic, and experimental care, on the one hand, and differences between purportedly objectively-grounded medical treatment and prevention on the other. Clinicians may bristle at the idea that they are engaged in a normative practice, preferring instead to view that practice as purely or mainly descriptive. Indeed, one great hope of medicine is that science will free us increasingly from subjectivity. In addition, the pursuit of objective standards can serve as psychological and rhetorical respite from the subjective nature of things—in short, a mechanism for the avoidance of politics.[42] As a presentation by the large private insurer UnitedHealthcare promises, "Based upon a foundation of evidence-based medicine, Medical Necessity is the process for determining benefit coverage and/or provider payment for services, tests, or procedures which are medically appropriate and cost-effective for the individual member."[43] At the base of the company's standards for evidence lies a commitment to "credible, published, scientific evidence supported by controlled clinical trials or observational studies." The company's evocation of evidence is intended to establish scientific grounds for its decision-making process while making clear that financial outcomes resulting from those decisions will be viewed as purely clinical decisions.

When one looks closely at the totality of medical evidence through the peer-reviewed literature of a given disease or condition, especially in systematic reviews, it becomes clear that the promise of evidence-based medicine is largely aspirational. At a minimum, the potential that evidence will resolve medical necessity disputes and disagreements is oversold. Without downplaying evidence-based medicine's potential, which I do believe is endless, I merely call attention to its unevenness as well as its persuasive role in medical necessity decision making. Thus, while Aetna's Clinical Policy Bulletin lists chiropractic, biofeedback, acupuncture, and electrical stimulation as covered services because they are supported in the peer-reviewed medical literature, therapies that have not received such scholarly support—such as acupressure, cupping, and dance therapy—are deemed experimental and investigational.[44] In many ways, of course, these examples are predictable. They may, it should be stated, simply be illegitimate forms of medical treatment, and my aim is not to defend the illegitimate, but to question the means by which legitimacy is bestowed. But when discourses of the legitimately medical are shot through with power, we must ask why one form of care is considered legitimate while another is not. Pointing to evidence is not sufficient to the degree that evidence itself is subject to important considerations of power itself.

There are other problems with turning to evidence as a way out of the medical necessity puzzle. As Rosenbaum and colleagues note, "By choosing a high evidentiary, or tightly limited, standard regarding the evidence that must be present in order to satisfy coverage eligibility, such as the evidence-based medicine standard of requiring two controlled, randomized clinical trials before a medical intervention can be proven effective, insurers could impose limits on many types of care."[45] The possibility of a certain mode of care being made available to a particular patient requires the funding and focus needed for randomized controlled trials to be performed in the first place, raising the specter of a catch-22 as concerns already marginalized treatments.

Layers of power are at work in constraining and enabling randomized controlled trials. The loop this effect establishes suggests that some interventions may lack trials for the same reason that practitioners and health insurers are skeptical of their efficacy. But even in the realm of mainstream medicine, profitability plays an important role. As Trisha Greenhalgh and colleagues have argued, "the drug and medical devices industries increasingly set the research agenda."[46] The prevalence of industry-sponsored research establishes pathways that lead all the way to medical necessity decision making.

While acknowledging the important contribution that elite forms of knowledge make to medical necessity, we cannot lose sight of the fact that scientific claims are no less discursive or contestable. It is for this reason that I have emphasized the importance of rhetorical analysis. Even the vaunted evidence that so many hope will provide a way out of the subjective is always part of a persuasive art. Contestability is often obscured by rhetorical effects designed precisely to accomplish this goal. Noticing how medical necessity's rhetorical structure is constructed—and acknowledging that it is constructed at all—carries with it an insurrectionary potential that can be a powerful tool for critically engaging with medical necessity.[47] This requires charting the qualitative moves that stakeholders make in the course of defining medical necessity.

Increasingly, with advocates of transparency in science gaining attention,[48] scientific evidence is being increasingly recognized as contextual, partial, and contingent. This should be a cause for celebration, instead of concern, just as acknowledging medical necessity's inherent openness should be viewed as an opportunity for clarity and improvement—and a chance to better understand how the institutions and political actors that shape medical necessity tend to "infuse [it] with value."[49] Acknowledging medical necessity's openness to critique and political contestation enables actors of various sorts to respond to and engage medical claims when they are governed by values that they might want to either reject, challenge, or accept only provisionally.

Given the trajectory that most medical necessity scholarship has taken, the centrality and unavoidability of norms seems a relatively basic but consequential finding. In contrast to the arguments advanced by scholars who have sought to evade medical necessity's normative dimensions, it appears increasingly clear that engaging with these dimensions is the important work that lies ahead. After all, as Jennifer Prah Ruger notes, the goal of improving the health of populations requires "invoking principles, values and norms, and honest discussions about the consequences of denying necessary and appropriate care for people's health and security."[50] Given the contentiousness of such conversations, this will be easier said than done. Ruger herself even appears to take "necessary and appropriate" to be relatively unproblematic terms while focusing on the consequences of providing, or not providing, such services. Perhaps most problematic is the fact that the avoidance of normative dimensions is itself a key component of the rhetorical structuring of the politics of medical necessity. For example, Sabin and Daniels believe that science may help mitigate medical necessity debates while acknowledging that "conflicts over effectiveness may not currently be resolvable because of limited outcomes data, but they will ultimately yield to scientific progress."[51] In so doing, they join those scholars who suggest that tailoring interventions to individuals will generate a more persuasive connection between interventions and medical necessity, once again attempting to circumvent the contentious politics of medical necessity debates themselves.

I am not so optimistic. First, the solution that advocates of this approach envision amounts to little more than the taking hold of a rhetoric of objectivity, underscoring and benefiting from objectivity's persuasive force. More than that, much is lost in the imagined objectivity, particularly civic and community-based engagement with the establishment of medical priorities, both of which require maintaining spaces for rhetorical critique and innovation. Instead of the promise of science, as traditionally understood, conflicts about medical necessity are often driven by disagreements over what is and what is not medical, the "*ends* of health care," and "the *means* to achieve those ends."[52] This makes sense insofar as the politics of medical necessity tends to not only concern disagreement, but does so at a high level of abstraction, as though broad theoretical commitments will make medical necessity more predictable and stable. As such, the politics are rarely concerned with the technical means to the ends. But the ends are precisely what should remain open for debate, since it is here that social values are most clearly deposited and affirmed.

The important question is the integrity of the scientific process itself, cast as a perennial commitment rather than an outcomes-based activity capable of settling or closing medical necessity debates. It is for this reason that Derrida associates openness of inquiry, and the incompleteness of knowledge and the language in which it is embedded, with justice.[53] One might also argue that the goal I am advocating contains a democratic commitment as well, though I also accord special value, as is appropriate, to forms of specialized knowledge and training. Clinicians are trained for a reason, and their voices should carry weight. So, too, should clinical trials and other foundations of clinical evidence be accorded respect and consideration. But to privilege those voices alone is to misunderstand what medicine and medical outcomes require. Even the most seemingly technical of questions in medicine are social.

Sabin and Daniels worry that if we do not undertake the difficult work of establishing standards for medical necessity decision making, then we will continue to default to arbitrary capping of health services. In a sense, I am criticizing not only the project of establishing such standards, but also the "we" of the process itself. In an increasingly neoliberal system in which econometric and actuarial sciences wield extraordinary power, scholars must respond to these forces' tendencies to privatize questions of social origin and importance. At the same time, it is unwise to respond to the arbitrariness of standards with alternative standards that are only differently arbitrary. The more important goal is to think in terms of the power to decide and of modes of representation and input instead of prescribed standards. In other words, explicitly political categories are important to keep at the forefront of deliberations. For purposes of appearing nonpolitical, of course, institutions and actors involved in medical necessity decision making avoid rhetoric that reveals normative argument. They seek, moreover, to suppress not only norms, but the presence of rhetoric itself; this rhetoric, when openly marked as rhetoric, tends to call attention to the norms that make arguments persuasive instead of merely pointing to reports of purportedly objective fact.[54] A critical point in this regard is that medical necessity is not only essentially contestable from a definitional perspective, but as a normative horizon as well, in terms of ends. This gives the concept its ethical relevance and political quality. This approach also recaptures the medicine-as-art aspect that many physicians support, where their judgment plays an important role in decision making.

To take this position is not, however, to suggest that medical necessity is purely normative, a product of perspective or self-interests. To the contrary, this appeal toward norms is intended to promote transparency and openness, including an acknowledgment that what is being defended is perspective rather than natural, objective, or fixed positions. American health care would be more open to critique if we could acknowledge that its approach to medicine is largely a function of choices, even though disagreements would likely be no less contentious. This could, however, move the discussion to the procedures and processes through which decision making occurs, and make the normative aspects of those procedures and processes known. At a minimum, this would require the increased regulation of insurance industry practices, which remain inscrutable and largely unknown to the average patient. In the vision I am advancing, the normative positions of insurers and other relevant professional organizations would also be available for scrutiny.

This move toward transparency is the strategy that Bloche advocates from his position of viewing medical necessity as a cover for "quiet" limit-setting. For Bloche, "the current regime of covert rationing, under cover of 'medical necessity,' should be supplanted by visible resource allocation rules—rules set for doctors and patients by social institutions."[55] To play on Bloche's language, the advocacy of a more open politics of medical necessity requires the unearthing or uncovering of the decision-making process. In this view, whether these limits are set via "cost-benefit trade-off principles applicable to all" (his preference) or through market mechanisms that produce winners and losers, they "must be done in the open."[56] Given the myriad problems associated with attempts to evade the politics of medical necessity, scholars must turn to processes for adjudicating and critiquing medical necessity decision making's normative basis, thereby working through the value sets that should govern it. Promoting transparency—especially in private companies, who continue to resist efforts to require that they reveal their internal mechanisms for deliberation—would be a critical step in this direction. This will become increasingly important as we engage controversial aspects of utilization review, such as the importance of carefully reviewing medical charts before issuing denials, as Aetna was recently exposed for failing to do, or Anthem's goal of establishing post facto review of emergency department utilization, especially imaging. In the case of the Anthem policies, hospital organizations have claimed that the fact that some hospitals have been offered exemptions if they accept lower reimbursement rates demonstrates that the policies are being implemented with clear disregard for medical necessity.[57] In their lawsuit against Anthem, the hospitals charge that the Anthem policies emphasize cost and "site of care" over clinical judgment. The latter reminds us that location plays an important role in the utilization review of health services.

A somewhat more radical alternative to simply acknowledging the role of norms would be to advocate a politics that gives greater weight to individual self-assertions of need, perhaps by cultivating respect for the ability to determine and declare one's needs in a comparatively un-restrained manner. This would, of course, put considerable pressure on, as well as meet considerable resistance from gatekeepers concerned pri-marily with moral hazard and financial bottom lines. However, individu-als are often at a disadvantage vis-à-vis institutionalized medical power. This is true in a number of ways. It is true, as we have discussed, with regard to asymmetric markets that place individuals in a position of epis-temic disadvantage when making decisions about health insurance and their own projected needs. It is also true with regard to the complexities of physician–patient and patient–system relationships, which are extraordi-narily difficult to rework in such a way that they truly empower patients. These challenges persist, despite decades of rhetoric about informed con-sent, patient choice, patient-centeredness, and the like. Affording greater weight to self-assertions of need would serve as a counterweight.

Though the pragmatics of such a position make it a largely unrealistic and problematic choice, it is worth noting that there may even be cases in which we could lift the threshold entirely. This would require taking seriously individual's claims about who they are and what they need, not only to survive, but to live flourishing lives characterized by an expansive notion of health. Such an approach would necessarily put pressure on bio-medical as well as neoliberal economic models. They would also require safeguards to ensure that informed consent does not function as a de facto tool for coercion by clinicians. However, in fleshing out our theory of such a position, it is important to note that while such a position would seem, at first, capable of significantly revising the power/knowledge sys-tems that currently govern medicine, this is not necessarily the case, to the extent that power/knowledge is maintained just as much by internalized norms as repressive forces seemingly operating from the outside. Such an approach would likely be met with intense resistance along conservative lines, with a predictably disproportionate level of scrutiny applied in po-litically charged areas, such as at the intersections of gender and sexuality. It is important to notice, however, that empowering individuals does not move us outside of social power and the discursive matrices that sustain it.

Another slightly more direct problem, of course, is that this emphasis on individual voices is unlikely to yield good health outcomes. There is considerable evidence that empowering patients is an important value in medical decision making,[58] but we must also acknowledge that patients often lack the technical and scientific know-how to make this ethical strategy worth defending in and of itself. Merely empowering patients to decide without providing them with tools for thinking critically about their situation is no better than affording physicians unchecked authority in medical decision making. Though it is clearly important that in future medical developments individual patients should be listened to more, it is also the case that individuals may make bad choices. The more important point resides in collaborative and team-based decision making, not only broadening the scope of possible voices (patients, physicians, social workers, clergy, and beyond), but—and this is the critical step—ensuring that those voices gain rhetorical traction and are afforded legitimacy. In other words, part of the problem with the politics of medical necessity may be that physicians often have *too much* authority, are trusted too much, and their patients trust them to a fault. Though this authority is attenuated in principle by institutions such as informed consent and even utilization review, not to mention the previously discussed circulation of information available on the internet, we know that it remains rhetorically powerful for patients.

While physicians and patients complain of the intrusion by external voices into their medical decision-making process, we are entering into a new era in which this dyadic focus is changing. An increasingly decentralized politics of medical necessity will need to value new stakeholders—actors who are genuinely committed to patient care and the pursuit of better outcomes—and not the autonomy of any one stakeholder. I thus join those who lament profit-driven counterweights to physicians' ability to determine medical necessity autonomously, as well as a blind faith in quality metrics that may or may not be appropriate or evidence based, while also underscoring the need to attenuate unilateral authority. Team-based care is undoubtedly the future of medicine; the key question concerns the expansiveness, quality, and logistics of enabling such a team to function effectively. This will also require taking on interest and pressure groups as part of this politics to ensure that their voices do not fill the outsized space they currently occupy. In this way, new norms can be established in a comparatively decentralized but still evidence-based manner, where evidence is derived not from one clinical corner, or one interest, but broad, consultative, and more humanistically informed quarters. To this extent, the politics of medical necessity mirrors that of other political questions, where contingency and predictability, liberty and autonomy and constraint and regulation, and elite and popular forms of knowledge must be balanced.

Engaging Politics

The AMA has boldly declared: "The standard for determining whether care is 'medically necessary' in a managed care setting has become an issue of national importance."[59] Though the heyday of managed care has waned, we are still in an era of management of a different sort. The key question is whether uncertainty about medical necessity will give rise to a broad-based or more even national politics.

To date, of course, this has not happened. This is because most people experience medical necessity in private, after having received a denial, often in the form of a bill. Though bills can become important pieces of larger journalist and activist efforts,[60] in their everydayness they rarely materialize into calls to civic action. Some of these stories make headlines, but most do not, and are dealt with in isolation or not dealt with at all. To this extent, the privatization and capitalization of medical experience is part of a neoliberal movement that an open politics could subvert, at least in part. Moreover, most denials are not the basis of an appeal, which means that medical necessity is rarely challenged, for complex reasons of patient knowledge and empowerment, time, as well as financial resources. In addition, we can assume appeals to cut across the same lines as other modes of recourse requiring support and resources, with minorities and the marginalized less likely to appeal than the empowered and privileged.

Precisely because so much medical decision making is privatized, dispersed within the file folders and ledger books of opaque institutions, the United States has evaded questions of medical necessity that countries with national health care system have, to varying degrees, undertaken.[61] In the United States, while rancorous discussions about health care utilization and best practices of Medicare and Medicaid have stimulated a number of national debates—particularly among physicians and professional advocacy groups—a broad national debate has yet to take hold. The forces that could lead to critical thinking about medical necessity are baked, often to a point of invisibility, into American health care policymaking itself. A critical politics of medical necessity requires that we show how various forces seek to shape medical necessity's conceptual contours for their own ends.

We must reclaim this act of boundary drawing as part of a political project that puts patients and populations first.

This resistance to directly engaging medical necessity is common even in the wake of large-scale health care reform, such as that the ACA introduced. Bluntly put, medical necessity was never on the legislative agenda.[62] In fact, the one attempt to apply some oversight and rethinking of priorities in the interest of the long-term solvency of Medicare—the Independent Payment Advisory Board (IPAB), which the ACA authorized—was long a central target of ACA critics who characterized it with many of the familiar rhetorical histrionics, from "death panels" to "rationing."[63] Though IPAB's statutory charge did include issuing recommendations that "protect and improve Medicare beneficiaries' access to necessary and evidence-based items and services,"[64] it was never authorized to address medical necessity. Rather than focusing on specific medical necessity protocols or contributing to a focused discussion of whether Medicare is construing medical necessity in an acceptable manner, IPAB was to make recommendations to Congress about system-level reforms to promote evidence-based practices. As such, IPAB—no doubt for political reasons—was forbidden to address two major elephants in the room: cost and how we construe need. IPAB's relative toothlessness is another example of how misaligned incentives, driven by major industry stakeholders, have prevented us from addressing some of the most critical questions hampering the development of a better American health care system. After years of controversy, IPAB was repealed as part of the Republican overhaul of the U.S. tax system.[65]

Beyond debates over strategies of cost containment and initiatives that support the pursuit of evidence-based medicine, it is clear more generally that the patchwork, Rube Goldberg nature of the American health care system has forestalled the kind of broad social deliberations over the meaning of medical necessity that tend to take hold in nations with universal national health care systems, where shared resources must be managed and negotiated. Each of these components is guarded jealously by the various interests that have a stake in maximizing profitability. As a result, in the American model these debates remain largely privatized, relegated to problems for individuals to grapple with and a government that is incapable and unwilling to take on the interest and pressure groups that ensure that the process remains lucrative. One need only look to the ACA for evidence of this dynamic, as the Obama administration's key move in even making expanded access to health insurance for millions of Americans possible was inviting major stakeholders—especially the pharmaceutical, insurance, and hospital industries—into negotiations. A predictable outcome of the horse trading that occurs within health policy is a lack of vibrant public discourse about any of most fundamental questions of what an acceptable health care system might look like. As a result, medical necessity decision making remains either hidden or difficult to unearth without legal and formal appeals. Complex appeals processes and lawsuits appear to be the standard, even primary American approach to unearthing medical necessity's theoretical contours and archival origins. Nonetheless, the initiation and navigation of these processes falls on the shoulders of individuals who must navigate them largely on their own.

Canada provides a useful contrast in this regard, as a commitment to universal health coverage has forced a debate over priorities. While far from perfect, compared to the United States' emphasis on market competition, the Canada Health Act's control over the provision of medically unnecessary health services is based on a belief that such provisions "erode the public system by destroying its broad base of support and increasing costs."[66] This policy is intended to remove the possibility that medical judgments might be made for purposes other than providing high quality, clinically sound care, but also to keep costs low so as to maintain the broader system.[67] In this regard, sustained engagement with the question of medical necessity is seen as a precondition of universal coverage, which again is rather unhelpfully called, in American rhetorical terms, "rationing." The result is comparatively broad social engagement with the process, as well as a greater critical eye on the procedural aspects through which health care utilization is regulated in the provinces. This approach forces Canadians to engage the question of medical necessity directly since (at least within provinces) universal standards create communal stakes regarding the definitions of key terms. In other words, universality forces broad deliberation. Just as importantly, universal health care tends to make visible the politics of access by forcing a political question about the social meanings of necessity.[68] Historically, trust in the government's role in these decision-making processes has tended to earn the support of a majority of Canadians, compared with a persistent distrust of their government by Americans.[69]

Universality, of course, does not solve the definitional problems associated with medical necessity. After all, as Baker and Bhabha succinctly put it, universality is a commitment on the side of access, and "has never meant coverage for everything."[70] In many ways, however, as I have suggested, universality plays an important role in forcing productive medical necessity debates. In Canada, for example,

> medical necessity is a contentious battleground in which citizens and government are locked in an interpretive struggle over the scope of this coverage, and the types of services deemed to be medically necessary. Disputes about medical necessity can arise when services that had previously been listed are delisted, whether based on "evidence-based" analysis, physician-government negotiations designed to respond to financial constraints or the political viewpoint of the government of the day. Alternatively, they may arise when a new treatment has been developed and remains to be decided whether or not its claim for recognition is warranted.[71]

In this case, medical necessity is evoked in the service of not only restricting care, but protecting the solvency of and public support for a system.[72] Yet, as Wennberg argues, despite the advantages for critically engaging medical necessity that national health systems offer, both Canada and the United States "have failed to confront the conundrum of what constitutes medical necessity and therefore our ability to identify when valuable care is being rationed."[73] While decisions about coverage priorities have been made within the various provinces, this has not led to a general theory for defining medical necessity.

A related step concerns the potential for groups who are similarly located to play a larger and collaborative role in establishing priorities in medical decision making—that is, to democratize the decision-making process by bringing group power to bear on it. In the United States, this may be helped along as traditional biomedical models give way, even if slowly, to population-based strategies of prevention and wellness. Particularly in the United States, where the consolidation of private health systems is producing, with increasing speed, megasystems that simultaneously generate formidable and likely intractable cultures of medical necessity decision making of their own, there may be a particularly auspicious opportunity for additional actors—including community-based nonprofits, faith-based groups, and beyond—to weigh in.[74] Under the ACA, nonprofit hospitals are tasked with soliciting community feedback that could include input about the structural boundaries of medical necessity, translating it into an explicitly community vernacular. These groups are well positioned to testify to the ways in which deeper structural issues at the heart of social justice and equality may precede the more fine-grained questions and structures that shape medical necessity decision making, based in part by their experiences in clinical spaces, but also as informants on the community level. After all, among other things, these structures set "the broad boundaries within which structural reforms to health care can take place."[75] Such boundaries are political, and remind us that certain aspects of the politics of medical necessity are functions of American institutions and the cultures they have shaped. They are historical productions; indeed, the politics of medical necessity I have mapped is part of a cultural inheritance of American health care politics itself.

These findings suggest the possibility of embracing a politics of medical necessity in which the term is understood as a signifier of value instead of a referent of "real" or "actual" necessity. This approach allows the rhetoric of medical necessity to continue to be part of a negotiation of health care utilization without the problematic significations that the term "rhetoric" evokes. Such a use would acknowledge that necessity can be deployed in different rhetorical registers, and that a multitude of actors can legitimately weigh in, even if the modifier "medical" skews the discourse toward clinicians. If medical necessity is best understood as a rhetoric of intertwined and overlapping shades of gray instead of the binary and mutually exclusive categories of black and white, there may be an opening for rethinking patients' access to care that lacks firm evidence, as much of it often does.

For example, care denied as "investigational" is increasingly being worked back into coverage in some private plans so long as it is part of a clinical trial, which could be of some benefit to terminal patients.[76] It may be that marijuana, stuck in the recreational–medical binary, could play a role in mitigating the opioid crisis by providing a safer alternative to opioids, like heroin or the deadly, and increasingly ubiquitous, synthetic drug fentanyl.[77] Medical necessity becomes a quite different discourse when viewed within fields of comparative risk instead of rhetorics of pure or uncomplicated necessity. Though we do not yet know if this would be the actual outcome, and must keep in mind that such studies are often limited in explanatory power,[78] it is worth exploring whether loosening restrictions around marijuana use may be a smart short-term policy in the face of a crisis that kills thousands each month. And, as the authors of recent studies emphasize, at a minimum the scale of the opioid crisis should persuade policy makers to fund and pursue research that could potentially help large numbers of Americans.

At the same time, without undermining these efforts, it should be acknowledged that the lack of marijuana research coupled with the vocal advocacy of promarijuana groups suggests that we remain skeptical as we encounter the medical necessity arguments that are likely to follow. Within this aspect of the politics of medical necessity it is worth asking, though it is difficult to answer for certain, whether marijuana advocates are advancing marijuana because they believe that it could actually have a tangible effect in weaning opioid users from opioids, or whether they are attaching their cause to a national crisis that has gained the attention of policy makers, average Americans, and beyond. Or perhaps the answer is both.

There is some precedent for using these rhetorical distinctions in such a strategic manner to creatively address important health challenges. Health services researcher Anna Tosteson distinguishes medical classifications for study purposes and those appropriate for intervention, with the assumption that a certain degree of medicalization is required for naming objects of study, while maintaining that such a classification should not carry the force associated with accessing medical care or insurance coverage. She argues, for example, that the term osteopenia was coined "mostly because they thought it might be useful for public health researchers who like clear categories for their studies." "They never imagined," she says, "that people would come to think of osteopenia as a disease in itself to be treated."[79] This marks a difference between researchers making a claim about the existence of osteopenia for research purposes—to secure funding, for example—and patients making treatment claims. The distinction attempts to restrict medical necessity's legal and social force to certain uses. Osteopenia is regarded not as a medical condition but a warning sign for possible osteoporosis, which licenses a series of medical interventions and necessity claims for which—under current norms—health insurance providers will pay. The notion of "prediabetes" operates similarly to osteopenia, serving less as a clinical indication or diagnosis than a persuasive framing to encourage patients to change their diets and other behaviors.[80] Rhetorical structures such as these suggest that the fact that a condition is named does not necessarily establish medical necessity, but also that there is a considerable gray area regarding the difference between degenerative conditions in progress and urgent or even chronic medical need.

The preceding chapters raise a question about whether medical necessity can or cannot, or should or should not, serve as a conceptual hinge point within the broader context of health promotion, as well as at the boundary of acute and chronic care. Debates about wellness, for example, raise questions about how to prevent situations of medical necessity from arising altogether, reducing the need for medical interventions as well as the cost of medical care. While medical necessity—taken at an extreme— signifies absolute need, the actual situations patients find themselves in may require a subtler vernacular, including distinctions made by social scientists between disease and illness,[81] as well as health, wellness, and flourishing. While there is often great variation in acute care decision making, chronic care introduces a more complex set of questions. These questions include problems concerning access to appropriate services, and an outdated approach to long-term care that fails to address needs, especially concerning limited function.[82] At the same time, health systems that emphasize preventive care are likely to require less care for chronic disease, lessening the need for medical necessity decision making altogether, or at least lowering the stakes of expanding the scope of medical necessity to include costly interventions.

Perhaps more to the point: should prevention be forced to travel under the sign of medical necessity at all? Only if we temper our expectations about the possibility of introducing newly depoliticized strategies for handling medical necessity does this make sense, to such an extent that the powerful rhetoric of medical necessity is often the only tool capable of guaranteeing access to care. Considering medical necessity's persistence, a more agonistic, assertive politics of medical necessity, pushed by vulnerable and underserved populations in need of care—whether acute or preventive—may be the only available or promising path. If we are to concede medical necessity's relative permanence in the rhetorical order of health care utilization then it is important that the broader point remains clear, namely that it will be necessary to scrutinize how, and with what ends, medical necessity determinations are made. This avenue of inquiry focuses less on medical necessity's definitional boundaries, or the pursuit of stable epistemic foundations within that definitional politics, and approaches medical necessity interpretation as an explicitly political practice. Such an approach would rework the very notion of necessity itself, not only as a limiting principle, but as a roadmap for building a health care system in which the justifications for health care utilization are established through clear processes in which a range of voices are heard. Various political traditions can agree on this fundamental point—from libertarian contractarians to progressives and social democrats who prefer the language of public health. Moving medical necessity from its currently individualized form to enable it to take on a more social character will be the challenge.

As one would expect, in advocating the politicization of medical necessity and subjecting it to critique, I position myself against a considerable consensus in the medical literature. Such an approach tends to make key stakeholders nervous, perhaps with good reason. For example, medical sociologist David Mechanic, in an important attempt to clarify myth and fact regarding public perceptions of managed care, notes that "much uncertainty in medical care remains, creating the need for a better understanding of how processes of care affect outcomes, and for evidence-based standards." This requires that managed care practices be fine-tuned "to evolve and become more sensitive to the many contingencies of people's lives." Yet, Mechanic also associates progress with the increased involvement of institutions that he sees as operating outside of politics, hence less subject to the corrosive effect of politics and public pressure. "Public trust," Mechanic declares, "is more likely to result from real accountability on the part of care providers than from political micromanagement."[83] Indeed, recent studies bear out the scope of the challenge facing medical professionals, as trust in medical institutions continues to decline.[84]

I quote Mechanic not to critique his commentary on trust, but because of how he characterizes politics, centered as it is on concerns such as "micromanagement" and the eclipsing of professional judgments by way of legislative intrusion. While it is of course possible, as Mechanic suggests, that available data does not always bear out the suspicions of managed care's critics, it is also true that managed care does not deserve any prima facie benefit of the doubt in the name of pursuing improved health outcomes.[85] Rather, if a large portion of American health care is to remain private, where transparency is not always a key commitment, truthfulness must be wrested from the forces—especially economic forces—that propel health care providers. Politics cannot be reduced to what legislators do. A more expansive conception is needed.

In fact, this lack of trust is one of the reasons I turn to rhetoric for thinking through the politics of medical necessity. There are a number of possible routes this turn could take. Enhancing the quality of communication

in the medical decision-making process is an important undertaking, especially insofar as it taps into rhetoric's traditional role in building con-
nections and finding points of mutual understanding.[86] This approach
underscores the consequences of pretending that cost-effectiveness is not
a major consideration in the allocation of health resources when, in fact,
it clearly and unavoidably is. Given the significance of cost to both individual patient care and challenges in the development and maintenance
of health care systems, it may be that the ultimate engagement with the
politics of necessity requires discussing cost, though this must be done
carefully, and in an ethical manner. It must be done not under the illu-
sion that we are tacking some absolute notion of medical necessity to the
financing of health care services, but that we are deciding along the way
what we wish to include under the malleable and normative umbrella of
necessity. The key political question, of course, is who this "we" is. Inclu-
sivity and nondiscrimination, as well as an aggressive and conscious effort
to engage marginalized peoples and communities, will be central to such a
plan being possible even in principle.

As Susan Miller has argued, the rhetorical structure of texts is essential
to building trust, not only from the top down in terms of observers' relations with elites, but in terms of being able to follow and participate in the
production of knowledge.[87] In paying close attention to the language
implicated in producing social perceptions and the legal codification of
medical necessity, I advocate a conception of medical necessity that even if
not true in a metaphysical sense, at least instills confidence in those most
impacted by it. This is different than Foucault's notion of being "within
the true," which he evokes to characterize the relationship of truth and
power within systems of power/knowledge.[88] Beyond being "in the true,"
it is more useful to follow Wittgenstein in his assertion that truth "is what
human beings say that is true and false; and they agree in the language
they use."[89] The key piece of this Wittgensteinian insight is agreement,
which requires that power be contested and exposed to such an extent—as
Foucault's entire oeuvre aimed to do—that patients and other stakeholders
can clearly see how social truths are constructed, and participate in their
reconstruction. A rhetorical reading amends the Wittgensteinian formu-
lation by adding: "and what is true is a matter of persuasion within language." This, as I have shown, is no mere duel between physicians and
patients, though it is sometimes also that. Beyond such dyadic duels there

is a vast network of persuasive forces circulating among clinical, social, economic, and other actors.

Medical necessity is, from this perspective, a contested *social* text rather than a purely technical or clinical matter. Trust between patients, physicians, and others must be sought despite the various suspicions that managed care has cast over the past decades.[90] All actors must be persuaded that decision making is being done reasonably and in good faith. Openly casting the process of decision making as one of competing interests rather than appeals to fixed points established by science would be a step in the right direction. Perhaps, if we are able to accomplish this, the more problematic rhetoric in health care debates—from rationing to death panels to socialism to rights—will be able to subside as a more civic-minded approach to medicine takes its place. There are, after all, more good-faith actors in American health care than observers tend to acknowledge. With this in mind, a broad range of voices can and must be activated and included to write medical necessity's boundaries. These boundaries will not always be appealing or even acceptable to elites.

At present, however, trust lies quite far afield, with longstanding suspicions compounded and seemingly confirmed by news reports of dubious practices by insurers. This lack of trust is palpable in both managed care and government insurance programs alike. In the 2016 presidential primary, critics of insurance companies spanned the political divide, from Ben Carson to Bernie Sanders. These forms of distrust are deeply embedded in American political culture itself, and are therefore unlikely to wane.[91] But it seems a missed opportunity to not emphasize the contingent status of American health care as we know it. A reconsideration of medical necessity is a key piece of rebuilding trust in medical systems and institutions. Accordingly, one of the goals of this book is to replace generalized trust in systems—and the definitional questions that comprise their daily work—with a more engaged politics precisely about the terms of medical care that Americans would like to see govern the system's various components. As regards medical necessity specifically, trust's utility is limited to the extent that it depoliticizes the terms of our medical care. The goal should be to develop systems that generate medical necessity arguments, and a general disposition toward medical necessity, that Americans can believe in, and to build institutions that can ensure that care is carried out with fidelity to those arrangements.

The problem is that trust in medical power lends support to uncritical ways of being. Unearned trust facilitates an understandable but nonetheless unacceptable wish that systems be free of normative content. For this reason, instead of trust I counsel healthy (but productive) skepticism—of physicians and other actors' judgments, as well as our own—as a way of attaining knowledge that is not the product of any one interest. The rhetorical approach I have advocated, which treats the politics of necessity as an engagement with contestable and interpretable texts, is a critical starting point.

Shedding light on and even embracing disagreement in medical politics of course comes at a cost. There will always be risk associated with disrupting existing pathways of legitimacy and power since they not only repress but call attention to the existing points of access, however problematic they may be. I have warned against simply pulling the medical necessity rug from under the most vulnerable Americans who depend upon its rhetorical power. But rethinking and reworking medical necessity in the interest of doing the work that is required of a twenty-first-century medicine will require that individuals wrestle with, rethink, and begin to disengage from the persuasive forces on which they have long depended.

The trade-off is worth making, though it must be done with care. After all, though it may sometimes be leveraged to secure care, the rhetoric of medical necessity can also be—and has been, as I have shown—used to disempower. The effect of such disempowerment could be the further loss of individual capacity to determine what one needs for oneself—and an expansion of unexamined deferment to external narratives and authorities. For this reason, the position I advocate would require the empowerment of traditionally marginalized groups in these conversations, from patients to communities to research institutions to a host of nontraditional actors that impact health. All of these stakeholders should participate in the process of attempting to better understand value and quality in health care. We should not expect the limited (and limiting) discourse of medical necessity to play a central role in creating a socially responsive health care system without at the same time situating that discourse in a significantly altered, more dynamic, and more critical political context.

Acknowledgments

A project that takes this long runs the risk of yielding an acknowledgment of tragicomic length. So, while I surely omit important names here, I acknowledge that friends, family, and colleagues from graduate school onward have all spurned, prodded, and encouraged me to finish this book. That said, a specific cast of characters has played particularly important roles.

Joan Tronto and Rosalind Petchesky were instrumental in shaping my early thinking about necessity in general, and medical necessity in particular. Both encouraged and supported me from graduate school into my early professional years, and continue to inspire my approach to and love of scholarly questions. I also acknowledge the support of many graduate school colleagues, especially Arthur Beckman, Jon Keller, Steve Pludwin, Patricia Stapleton, and Alex Zamalin. A special thanks goes to Jen Gaboury, who first convinced me, way back in 2007, that medical necessity was an important question about which I might have something worthwhile to say.

I am also grateful to colleagues I have had along the way, especially Jeremy Teigen (at Ramapo College), Tom Christenson, Monica Mueller, and David Summers (at Capital University), and many colleagues at Ohio University, especially Andrea Brunson, Berkeley Franz, Maureen McCann, Kyle Rosenberger, and Jackie Wolf. Nathaniel Powell provided critical research assistance that unearthed the intersections of medical necessity and marijuana for chapter 4. Jory Gomes read and provided feedback on the entire manuscript, catching mistakes and improving it with each read.

Pieter Martin, senior acquisitions editor at the University of Minnesota Press, took an early interest in this project and hung with me through rounds of reviews and complete overhauls of the manuscript. In a similar vein, I thank the various anonymous readers who gave their time and critical eye to this project. Though a multistage review process can be frustrating at times, the book is undeniably better for it. I'm also appreciative to Mary Russell, whose sharp eye and top-notch copyediting skill has greatly improved this manuscript's clarity and readability. I'll add: university presses are special places and I'm honored to be publishing with one of the great ones.

I'm lucky to have a loving family who supports my protracted scholarly projects. Were they still with us, I'm sure that my father, Charles Skinner, and my brother, Michael Skinner, would have been among this book's first readers, if not loyal critics. My mother, Alana Skinner, has been a rock of support through the process, as has my aunt Marianne "Bunny" Fohn; my sister-in-law Helena Fredriksson; and my nephew Otis Skinner.

My greatest appreciation must of course be reserved for Emily Taylor, a terrific and endlessly patient partner, and our four-year-old, Zebulon. Zeb, it should be known, has had to bear the brunt of my critical thinking about the rhetoric of necessity—which toddlers instinctively grasp as a stronger appeal than the rhetoric of wants, particularly where sweets and toys are concerned. It was when I heard Zeb tell his daycare friends that "my Daddy works in a coffee shop"—where I have spent hours upon hours completing this book—that I knew it was time to wrap this up and send the book to press.

Notes

Introduction

1. The rhetoric of medical necessity operates in the spirit of Wittgenstein's critique of time, which distinguished natural language use from philosophy. For Wittgenstein time was "something that we know when no one asks us, but no longer know when we are supposed to give an account of it." Ludwig Wittgenstein, *Philosophical Investigations: The German Text, with a Revised English Translation,* trans. G. E. M. Anscombe, 3rd ed. (Malden: Blackwell, 2003), sec. 89.

2. Samantha Raphelson, "Anthem Policy Discouraging 'Avoidable' Emergency Room Visits Faces Criticism," *NPR,* May 23, 2018.

3. Gallup, "Confidence in Institutions," http://news.gallup.com/poll/1597/confidence-institutions.aspx.

4. Dhruv Khullar, "Do You Trust the Medical Profession?" *New York Times,* January 23, 2018.

5. Wayne Drash, "Aetna Inquiry Widens over Ex-Medical Director's Comments," CNN.com, February 16, 2018.

6. Gerald W. Rothacker, "Hip and Knee Replacements Not So Readily Obtained Now," *LancasterOnline,* February 14, 2015.

7. CMS, "Documenting Medical Necessity for Major Joint Replacement (Hip and Knee)," *MLN Matters* SE1236, http://www.cms.gov/.

8. David Goldhill, *Catastrophic Care: Why Everything We Think We Know about Health Care Is Wrong* (New York: Vintage Books, 2013).

9. If anything, Trump-era reforms could tighten the strings. Or, if Americans lose health care coverage through a repeal bill, they will be forced to operate, to the extent that they can, in a cash-and-carry environment where insurance companies have little power over them, but they are likely to fail to receive care when they cannot pay.

10. David C. Cone et al., "Developing Research Criteria to Define Medical Necessity in Emergency Medical Services," *Prehospital Emergency Care* 8, no. 2 (2004): 116–25.

11. Maria C. Raven et al., "Comparison of Presenting Complaint vs Discharge Diagnosis for Identifying 'Nonemergency' Emergency Department Visits," *JAMA* 309, no. 11 (2013): 1145–53.

12. See Edward Melnick and Erik Hess, "How Shared Decision Making in the Emergency Department Can Improve Value," *Health Affairs Blog*, February 7, 2017.

13. Didier Fassin and Estelle D'Halluin, "The Truth from the Body: Medical Certificates as Ultimate Evidence for Asylum Seekers," *American Anthropologist* 107, no. 4 (2005): 597–608.

14. As just one example, recent reports suggest that unscrupulous businesses, acting in concert with predatory lenders, may stoke women's fears that they are in danger after having received vaginal mesh implants, leading to sometimes dangerous and unnecessary surgery. Matthew Goldberg and Jessica Silver-Greenberg, "How Profiteers Lure Women into Often-Unneeded Surgery," *New York Times*, April 14, 2018.

15. E. A. Jacobs et al., "Understanding African Americans' Views of the Trustworthiness of Physicians," *Journal of General Internal Medicine* 21, no. 6 (2006): 642–47.

16. On compliance, see Daniel Skinner and Berkeley Franz, "From Patients to Populations: Rhetorical Considerations for a Post-Compliance Medicine," *Rhetoric of Health & Medicine* 1, no. 3–4 (2019): 239–68. On malpractice and physician-patient communication, see J. Nguyen et al., "Communication-Related Allegations against Physicians Caring for Premature Infants," *Journal of Perinatology* 37, no. 10 (2017): 1148.

17. Foucault: "Power must be analyzed as something that circulates . . . it is never localised here or there, never in anybody's hands, never appropriated as a commodity or piece of wealth." Michel Foucault, *Power/Knowledge: Selected Interviews and Other Writings, 1972–1977*, ed. Colin Gordon (Brighton: Harvester Press, 1980), 98.

18. Many if not most books on rhetoric take this insight as a starting point. This includes Judy Z. Segal's path-breaking book, *Health and the Rhetoric of Medicine* (Carbondale: Southern Illinois University Press, 2005).

19. See Plato, *The Republic*, trans. Henry Desmond Pritchard Lee, 2nd ed., Penguin Classics (London: Penguin Books, 2003), Book I.

20. Foucault, *Power/Knowledge*, 81.

21. Raymie E. McKerrow, "Foucault's Relationship to Rhetoric," *The Review of Communication* 11, no. 4 (2011): 253–71. One must do this, however, while taking into account Foucault's concern to not conflate "discourse" and "rhetoric," the latter of which he "reserved for that kind of discourse that Plato disparaged so eloquently." Luanne Frank, "Michel Foucault," in *Twentieth-Century Rhetorics and Rhetoricians: Critical Studies and Sources*, ed. M. G. Moran and M. Ballif (Westport, Conn.: Greenwood Press, 2000), 172. Famously, Plato's distinction between rhetoric and philosophy is developed in his *Gorgias* dialogue.

22. McKerrow, "Foucault's Relationship to Rhetoric," 256.

23. McKerrow, 256.

24. Daniel Skinner, "The Politics of Medical Necessity in American Abortion Debates," *Politics & Gender* 8, no. 1 (2012): 1–24.

25. Jennifer Prah Ruger, *Health and Social Justice* (Oxford: Oxford University Press, 2009). The language comes from debates over constitutional interpretation. See Howard Lee McBain, *The Living Constitution: A Consideration of the Realities and Legends of Our Fundamental Law* (New York: Workers Education Bureau Press, 1927).

26. Johnnie St. Vrain, "An Arm and a Leg for an Eye and Tooth?," *Longmont Times-Call,* May 15, 2011, http://www.timescall.com.

27. Kenyon Wallace, "Newfoundland Denies Man 'Medically Necessary' Skin-Removal Surgery after 200-Pound Weight Loss," *Toronto Star*, January 17, 2012. As bariatric surgery becomes more common, we are also learning that patients are subject to an elevated risk of developing postsurgical skin conditions, many of which result from conditions caused by excess skin. See Ali Halawi, Firass Abiad, and Ossama Abbas, "Bariatric Surgery and Its Effects on the Skin and Skin Diseases," *Obesity Surgery* 23, no. 3 (2013): 408–13.

28. Bennett Hall, "Medical Mistake Claim against Good Sam Dropped," *Corvallis Gazette-Times,* May 15, 2012.

29. H. May Spitz, "Disabilities Act Outlines Rights, So Get Armed with Information," *Los Angeles Times,* February 18, 2007; Ken Amaro, "Resident Status Takes Bite Out of Fight to Keep Therapy Dog," *First Coast News*, January 12, 2012; and Rebecca J. Huss, "No Pets Allowed: Housing Issues and Companion Animals," *Animal Law Review* 22 (2005).

30. Matthew Waller, "Jeffs Leaves Hospital, Heads to Prison Infirmary," *Standard Times of San Angelo,* September 20, 2011.

31. George J. Annas, Sondra S. Crosby, and Leonard H. Glantz, "Guantanamo Bay: A Medical Ethics–Free Zone?," *New England Journal of Medicine* 369 (2013): 101–3.

32. Dominic Rushe et al., "Rectal Rehydration and Waterboarding: The CIA Torture Report's Grisliest Findings," *The Guardian*, December 11, 2014.

33. David Goldhill, *Catastrophic Care: Why Everything We Think We Know about Health Care Is Wrong* (New York: Vintage Books, 2013), xvi.

34. Goldhill, xvi.

1. Medical Necessity?

1. See James Crosswhite, "Universality in Rhetoric: Perelman's Universal Audience," *Philosophy & Rhetoric* 22, no. 3 (1989): 157–73.

2. Kinross, Robin, "The Rhetoric of Neutrality," *Design Issues* 2, no. 2 (1985): 18–30.

3. Raymond Williams, *Culture and Materialism: Selected Essays*, new ed. (New York: Verso, 2005), 67.

4. Michel Foucault, "The Order of Discourse," in *Language and Politics*, ed. Michael Shapiro (New York: New York University Press, 1984).

5. Sara Singer and Linda Bergthold, "Prospects for Improved Decision-Making about Medical Necessity," *Health Affairs* 20, no. 1 (2001): 205.

6. Cathy Charles et al., "Medical Necessity in Canadian Health Policy: Four Meanings and . . . a Funeral?," *The Milbank Quarterly* 75, no. 3 (1997): 365–94.

7. E. Haavi Morreim, "The Futility of Medical Necessity," *Regulation* 24, no. 2 (2001): 23.

8. Michael F. Cannon, "There Is No Objective Definition of 'Medical Necessity,'" *Cato at Liberty* (2012), http://www.cato.org/blog/there-no-objective-definition-medical-necessity.

9. Wittgenstein, *Philosophical Investigations*, sec. 241.

10. Wittgenstein and Foucault agree on this point. Where they depart significantly is on the nature of language games themselves, which Foucault would undoubtedly recast in terms of the decentralized power relations that govern them. Wittgenstein, as a language philosopher who rarely waded into politics in his scholarly work, does not offer tools for resolving these questions.

11. Charles et al., *Medical Necessity in Canadian Health Policy*, 386.

12. "Although our aggregate results confirm the utility of the concept of necessity, the lack of consensus among panelists on the necessity of indications is somewhat troubling." James P. Kahan et al., "Measuring the Necessity of Medical Procedures," *Medical Care* 32, no. 4 (April 1994): 357–65.

13. Peter A. Glassman, Peter D. Jacobson, and Steven Asch, "Medical Necessity and Defined Coverage Benefits in the Oregon Health Plan," *American Journal of Public Health* 87, no. 6 (1997): 1054.

14. Morreim, "The Futility of Medical Necessity," 22.

15. Linda A. Bergthold, "Medical Necessity: Do We Need It?," *Health Affairs* 14, no. 4 (1995): 182.

16. Bergthold, 181–82.

17. Daniel Knoepflmacher, "'Medical Necessity' in Psychiatry: Whose Definition Is It Anyway?" *Psychiatric News*, September 14, 2016.

18. Bergthold, "Medical Necessity," 182.

19. Heather Lyu et al., "Overtreatment in the United States," *PLOS ONE* 12, no. 9 (2017): e0181970.

20. Charles B. Hammond, "The Decline of the Profession of Medicine," *Obstetrics & Gynecology* 100, no. 2 (2002): 221–25.

21. Timothy S. Jost and Mark A. Hall, "The Role of State Regulation in Consumer-Driven Health Care," *American Journal of Law & Medicine* 31 (2005): 417. See also Mark A. Hall, "Institutional Control of Physician Behavior," *University of Pennsylvania Law Review* 137, no. 2 (1988): 431–536; J. B. McKinlay and L. D. Marceau, "The End of the Golden Age of Doctoring," *International Journal of Health Services* 32, no. 2 (2002): 379–416; D. W. Light, "The Medical Profes-

sion and Organizational Change: From Professional Dominance to Countervailing Power," in *Handbook of Medical Sociology*, ed. C. E. Bird, P. Conrad, and A. M. Fremont (Upper Saddle River, N.J.: Prentice Hall, 2000).

22. American Medical Association, "Model Managed Care Contract," sec. 1.11, 42.

23. Sara Rosenbaum et al., "Who Should Determine When Health Care Is Medically Necessary?," *New England Journal of Medicine* 340, no. 3 (1999): 229.

24. Bergthold, "Medical Necessity," 184.

25. William Sage, "Managed Care's Crimea: Medical Necessity, Therapeutic Benefit, and the Goals of Administrative Process in Health Insurance," *Duke Law Journal* 53, no. 2 (2003): 600.

26. Michel Foucault, *The History of Sexuality, Volume 1: An Introduction* (New York: Vintage Books, 1980).

27. Linda L. Layne, "'How's the Baby Doing?' Struggling with Narratives of Progress in a Neonatal Intensive Care Unit," *Medical Anthropology Quarterly* 10, no. 4 (December 1996): 639.

28. Glassman, Jacobson, and Asch, "Medical Necessity and Defined Coverage Benefits," 1054–55.

29. David H. Souter and the Supreme Court of the United States, *U.S. Reports: Pegram et al. v. Herdrich*, 530 U.S. 211 (2000), https://www.loc.gov/item/usrep530211/.

30. American Medical Association, *Model Managed Care Contract: Supplement 1*, "Medical Necessity and Due Process" (2005), http://www.montgomerymedicine.org.

31. John D. Lantos, *The Lazarus Case: Life-and-Death Issues in Neonatal Intensive Care* (Baltimore: Johns Hopkins University Press, 2001), 4.

32. See Stephen C. Shannon et al., "A New Pathway for Medical Education," *Health Affairs* 32, no. 11 (2013), which discusses the Blue Ribbon Commission for the Advancement of Osteopathic Medical Education's call for "new, team-based expertise to address the complexity of care needs."

33. Jonathan B. Imber, *Trusting Doctors: The Decline of Moral Authority in American Medicine* (Princeton, N.J.: Princeton University Press, 2008).

34. Harry P. Selker, "Capitated Payment for Medical Care and the Role of the Physician," *Annals of Internal Medicine* 124, no. 4 (1996): 449–51.

35. Glassman, Jacobson, and Asch, "Medical Necessity and Defined Coverage Benefits," 1055.

36. Glassman, Jacobson, and Asch, 1056.

37. Lantos, *The Lazarus Case*, 6.

38. Lantos, 6.

39. Derrick Augustus Carter, "Knight in the Duel with Death: Physician Assisted Suicide and the Medical Necessity Defense," *Villanova Law Review* 41, no. 3 (1996): 663–724.

40. John E. Wennberg, *Tracking Medicine: A Researcher's Quest to Understand Health Care* (Oxford: Oxford University Press, 2010), 253.

41. See, for example, Ana I. Balsa et al., "Clinical Uncertainty and Healthcare Disparities," *American Journal of Law and Medicine* 29, no. 2–3 (2003): 203–19.

42. Shedra Amy Snipes et al., "Is Race Medically Relevant? A Qualitative Study of Physicians Attitudes about the Role of Race in Treatment Decision-Making," *BMC Health Services Research* 11, no. 1 (2011): 6.

43. Paul Starr, *The Social Transformation of American Medicine* (New York: Basic Books, 1982).

44. "Direct-to-Consumer Advertising under Fire," *Bulletin of the World Health Organization* 87, no. 8 (2009); Bill Hendrick, "Self-Diagnosis from TV Drug Ads Can Be Dangerous," *Atlanta Journal-Constitution*, January 8, 2007.

45. Peter Elkind, Jennifer Reingold, and Doris Burke, "Inside Pfizer's Palace Coup," *Fortune,* August 15, 2011.

46. Simon J. Williams and Michael Calnan, "The 'Limits' of Medicalization?: Modern Medicine and the Lay Populace in 'Late' Modernity," *Social Science & Medicine* 42, no. 12 (1996): 1609–20.

47. K. Gogineni et al., "Patient Demands and Requests for Cancer Tests and Treatments," *JAMA Oncology*, no. 1 (2015): 33–39.

48. See, e.g., Jason Schnittker and Valerio Bacak, "The Increasing Predictive Validity of Self-Rated Health," *PLOS ONE* 9, no. 1 (2014): e84933.

49. Brian S. Alper, "Curbside Consultation: Usefulness of Online Medical Information," *American Family Physician* 74, no. 3 (2006).

50. Segal, *Health and the Rhetoric of Medicine*, 143.

51. Richard L. Kravitz et al., "Influence of Patients' Requests for Direct-to-Consumer Advertised Antidepressants: A Randomized Controlled Trial," *JAMA* 293, no. 16 (2005): 1995–2002.

52. James D. Reschovsky and Cynthia B. Saiontz-Martinez, "Malpractice Claim Fears and the Costs of Treating Medicare Patients: A New Approach to Estimating the Costs of Defensive Medicine," *Health Services Research* (2017).

53. Lantos, *The Lazarus Case*, 85.

54. Bridget M. Kuehn, "Patient-Centered Care Model Demands Better Physician-Patient Communication," *JAMA* 307, no. 5 (2012): 441–42.

55. Romana Hasnain-Wynia, "Is Evidence-Based Medicine Patient-Centered and Is Patient-Centered Care Evidence-Based?," *Health Services Research* 41, no. 1 (2006): 1.

56. Cited in Wendy Levinson, Cara S. Lesser, and Ronald M. Epstein, "Developing Physician Communication Skills for Patient-Centered Care," *Health Affairs* 29, no. 7 (2010): 1310–18.

57. Wennberg, *Tracking Medicine*, 64.

58. Wennberg, 65.

59. See, for example, "Topic Spotlight: Shared Decision Making," Patient-Centered Outcomes Research Institute, https://www.pcori.org/research-results/topics/shared-decision-making. According to PCORI's website, as of October 2017 the institute had funded 124 studies related to shared decision making and the development of decision tools.

60. Annemarie Mol, "Freedom or Socks: Market Promises versus Supportive Care in Diabetes Treatment," in Cindy Patton, ed., *Rebirth of the Clinic: Places and Agents in Contemporary Health Care* (Minneapolis: University of Minnesota Press, 2010), 109.

61. Henry T. Ireys, Elizabeth Wehr, and Robert E. Cooke, "Defining Medical Necessity: Strategies for Access to Quality Care for Persons with Developmental Disabilities, Mental Retardation, and Other Special Health Care Needs" (Baltimore: National Policy Center for Children with Special Health Care Needs, School of Hygiene and Public Health, the Johns Hopkins University, 1999), 29.

62. Sara Rosenbaum et al., "Medical Necessity in Private Health Plans: Implications for Behavioral Health Care," U.S. Department of Health and Human Services, Special Report, November 2003, 9. At https://hsrc.himmelfarb.gwu.edu/sphhs_policy_facpubs/171/.

63. Paul Chodoff, "Medical Necessity and Psychotherapy," *Psychiatric Services* 49, no. 11 (1998): 1481–83; William Ford, "Medical Necessity: Its Impact in Managed Mental Health Care," *Psychiatric Services* 49, no. 2 (1998): 183–84; and William Ford, "Medical Necessity and Managed Psychiatric Care," *Psychiatric Clinics of North America* 23, no. 2 (2000): 309–17.

64. Peter Conrad and Valerie Leiter, "Medicalization, Markets and Consumers," *Journal of Health and Social Behavior* 45 (2004): 170–71.

65. *Pegram*, 7.

66. Ireys, Wehr, and Cooke, "Defining Medical Necessity," 19.

67. *Pegram*, 22.

68. William Wagner, "Confronting Utilization Review in New Mexico's Medicaid Mental Health System: The Critical Role of 'Medical Necessity,'" *Medical Anthropology Quarterly* 19, no. 1 (2005): 79.

69. Pennsylvania Health Law Project, "Getting Patients What They Need: Appeals & Letters of Medical Necessity," http://www.phlp.org.

70. Aaron Seth Kesselheim, "What's the Appeal? Trying to Control Managed Care Medical Necessity Decision-Making through a System of External Appeals," *University of Pennsylvania Law Review* 149, no. 3 (2001): 873–920.

71. See Center for Medicare and Medicaid Services, Center for Consumer Information & Insurance Oversight, "External Appeals," https://www.cms.gov/cciio/Programs-and-Initiatives/Consumer-Support-and-Information/External-Appeals.html.

72. Center for Medicare and Medicaid Services, Center for Consumer Information & Insurance Oversight, "HHS-Administered Federal External Review Process for Health Insurance Coverage," https://www.cms.gov.

73. Sage, "Managed Care's Crimea," 599.

74. Lee N. Newcomer, "Who Should Determine When Health Care Is Medically Necessary?," *New England Journal of Medicine* 341 (1999): 58–60.

75. Patient Protection and Affordable Care Act, Pub. L. No. 111–148, § 2719, 124 Stat. 119, 318–319 (2010), https://www.congress.gov/111/plaws/publ148/PLAW-111publ148.pdf.

76. Patient Protection and ACA, 42 U.S.C. § 18001 (2010), section 1101(f). https://www.law.cornell.edu/uscode/text/42/18001.

77. Robert Pear, "New Medicare Rule Authorizes 'End-of-Life' Consultations," *The New York Times*, October 30, 2015.

78. Paula Span, "A Quiet End to the 'Death Panels' Debate," *New York Times*, November 20, 2015.

79. See, for example, Aetna, "Process for Disputes and Appeals," http://www.aetna.com.

80. Utilization Review Accreditation Commission, "URAC Releases Revised Independent Review Organization Standards," December 30, 2010, https://www.urac.org/news/urac-releases-revised-independent-review-organization-standards.

81. Sara Rosenbaum, Joel B. Teitelbaum, and Katherin J. Hayes, "The Essential Health Benefits Provisions of the ACA: Implications for People with Disabilities," *Realizing Health Reform's Potential* 3 (2011): 5.

82. Vernellia R. Randall, "Racist Health Care: Reforming an Unjust Health Care System to Meet the Needs of African-Americans," *Health Matrix* 3, no. 27 (1993), http://scholarlycommons.law.case.edu/healthmatrix/vol3/iss1/6.

83. Sara Rosenbaum, "The Americans with Disabilities Act in a Health Care Context," in *The Future of Disability in America*, ed. by M. J. Field and A. M. Jette (Washington, D.C.: National Academies Press, 2007).

2. In the Archive

1. Jacques Derrida, *Archive Fever: A Freudian Impression*, trans. E. Prenowitz (Chicago: University of Chicago Press, 1995).

2. To this extent, medical necessity determinations are both freed and riddled by Derrida's notion of *différence*—the deferral of meaning, which his analytic method of deconstruction seeks to chart. See *Writing and Difference* (Chicago: University of Chicago Press, 1978).

3. Michel Foucault, *The Birth of the Clinic*, trans. A. M. Sheridan Smith (New York: Vintage, 1994).

4. See Lisa Diedrich, "Practices of Doctoring," in Patton, *Rebirth of the Clinic*.

5. Patricia Aalseth, *Medical Coding: What It Is and How It Works* (Sudbury, Mass.: Jones & Bartlett Learning, 2005), 123.

6. Aalseth, 124.

7. American Medical Association Model Managed Care Contract: Supplement 6, "Downcoding and Bundling of Claims: What Physicians Need to Know About These Payment Problems," archived at http://www.scribd.com/doc/6437334/Downcoding-and-Bundling-Claims.

8. Foucault, *Birth of the Clinic*, 108.

9. T. M. Luhrmann, *Of Two Minds: An Anthropologist Looks at American Psychiatry* (New York: Vintage, 2001), 83.

10. Huynh Kyle, Joseph Grubbs, and Richard M. Davis, "An Eye for the Eye: *Seeing* Art in Medicine," *Journal of General Internal Medicine* 29, no. 3 (2014): 547–48.

11. Jane Macnaughton, "Medical Humanities' Challenge to Medicine," *Journal of Evaluation in Clinical Practice* 17, no. 5 (2011): 927–32.

12. See Judith H. Hibbard and Jessica Greene, "What the Evidence Shows about Patient Activation: Better Health Outcomes and Care Experiences; Fewer Data on Costs," *Health Affairs* 32, no. 2 (2013): 207–14.

13. Aalseth, *Medical Coding*, 1.

14. J. William Thomas, Erika C. Ziller, and Deborah A. Thayer, "Low Costs of Defensive Medicine, Small Savings from Tort Reform," *Health Affairs* 29, no. 9 (2010).

15. World Health Organization, International Classification of Diseases, http://www.who.int/classifications/icd/en.

16. American Medical Association, "Preparing for the ICD-10 Code Set: Fact Sheet 2," September 25, 2012. https://www.ama-assn.org/sites/ama-assn.org/files/corp/media-browser/premium/washington/icd10-icd9-differences-fact-sheet_0.pdf.

17. Terry Eagleton, *Literary Theory: An Introduction* (Malden, Mass.: Blackwell, 2008), 148.

18. Gary Greenberg, *The Book of Woe: The DSM and the Unmaking of Psychiatry* (New York: Blue Rider Press, 2012), 33.

19. Lisa Cosgrove et al., "Financial Ties between DSM-IV Panel Members and the Pharmaceutical Industry," *Psychotherapy and Psychosomatics* 75, no. 3 (2006): 154–60.

20. Deborah Kelly-Farwell and Cecile Favreau, *Coding for Medical Necessity in the Physician's Office: An In-Depth Approach to Record Abstracting* (Clifton Park, N.Y.: Cengage Learning, 2008).

21. Kelly-Farwell and Favreau, 113.

22. Luhrmann, *Of Two Minds*, 31.

23. Carolyn Long Engelhard, "Is Direct Primary Care Part of the Solution or Part of the Problem?," *The Hill,* October 13, 2014, 71. To avoid the DSM's imposition,

Greenberg's solution is "not to do business with insurance companies," a decision which he characterizes as "buying my way out of bad faith."

24. Aalseth, *Medical Coding*, 108–9.

25. "Sample Letter of Medical Necessity," BotoxReimbursementSolutions.com, https://www.botoxreimbursement.us/Resources/lmn.doc.

26. See P. J. Cloud-Moulds, "Medical Necessity: Physicians Need to Prove It to Payers," http://www.physicianspractice.com/blog/medical-necessity-physicians -need-prove-it-payers.

27. See, e.g., Michael J. Barry and Susan Edgman-Levitan, "Shared Decision-Making: The Pinnacle of Patient-Centered Care," *New England Journal of Medicine* 366 (2012): 780–81.

28. Aalseth, *Medical Coding*, 84, 133.

29. Aalseth (143–44) gives the following example: "According to official diagnosis coding guidelines, when a patient has a urinary tract infection, that code is sequenced first, before the code for the organism. If the order of the codes is switched, a higher weight DRG is assigned. If all the cases of this type in a hospital were sequenced improperly, that facility might be charged with intentional fraud."

30. Allied Health Schools, "10 Reasons to Become a Medical Biller or Coder," https://www.allalliedhealthschools.com/medical-billing-coding/medical-coding -career-reasons/.

31. Aalseth, *Medical Coding*, 158.

32. Marc Berg and Geoffrey Bowker, "The Multiple Bodies of the Medical Record: Toward a Sociology of an Artifact," *Sociological Quarterly* 38, no. 3 (1997): 513–37.

33. Foucault, *Birth of the Clinic*. See also Bruno Latour, *Science in Action: How to Follow Scientists and Engineers through Society* (Cambridge, Mass.: Harvard University Press, 1987).

34. Aalseth, *Medical Coding*, 109.

35. Kelly-Farwell and Favreau, *Coding for Medical Necessity*, 107.

36. Kelly-Farwell and Favreau, 108.

37. This points to the rhetorical notion of *kairos*, marked by Thomas Moore's expression, "This is the right time, and this is the right thing." At the same time, beyond time, kairos emphasizes location. For a discussion of rhetoric and the temporal/locational dimensions of situations, see Lloyd F. Bitzer, "The Rhetorical Situation," in *Rhetoric: Concepts, Definitions, Boundaries*, ed. by William A. Covino (Boston: Allyn and Bacon, 1995).

38. Carol Spencer, "Top Reason for RAC Denials: Lack of Medical Necessity in Wrong Setting," *RAC Monitor* (June 1, 2011), http://www.healthcarefinancenews .com.

39. Aalseth, *Medical Coding*, 111.

40. Michel Foucault, *Discipline and Punish: The Birth of the Prison* (New York: Vintage Books, 1979).

41. In a double sense. On the one hand, passing entails conforming to a norm. On the other, it entails not being noticed as a result of conforming to a norm.

42. Laura Dyrda, "8 Factors Impacting Spine Surgery Coverage Rates," *Becker's ASC Review* (March 7, 2013), http://www.beckersasc.com.

43. Douglas J. Jorgensen, "OMT Coding Strategies to Boost Your Bottom Line," *American Congress of Osteopathic Family Physicians*, archived at http://www.acofp .org.

44. Inga Ellzey, "Coding for Shave Removals vs. Biopsies," *The Dermatologist*, https://www.the-dermatologist.com/article/8857.

45. This was Plato's concern in the *Phaedrus*: "When it has once been written down, every discourse roams about everywhere, reaching indiscriminately those with understanding no less than those who have no business with it, and it doesn't know to whom it should speak and to whom it should not. And when it is faulted and attacked unfairly, it always needs its father's support; alone, it can neither defend itself nor come to its own support." Plato, *Complete Works*, edited by John M. Cooper and D. S. Hutchinson (Indianapolis: Hackett, 1997), 552.

46. See Rosalind P. Petchesky, *Abortion and Woman's Choice: The State, Sexuality, and Reproductive Freedom*, rev. ed. (Boston: Northeastern University Press, 1990).

47. John D. Lantos, *The Lazarus Case: Life-and-Death Issues in Neonatal Intensive Care* (Baltimore: Johns Hopkins University Press, 2001), 7.

48. This is not much different than the conditions of emergency and intensive care generally. See Tim Wenham and Alison Pittard, "Intensive Care Unit Environment," *Continuing Education in Anaesthesia, Critical Care, and Pain* 9, no. 6 (2009): 178–83.

49. Stanley Fish, *Doing What Comes Naturally: Change, Rhetoric, and the Practice of Theory in Literary and Legal Studies* (Durham, N.C.: Duke University Press, 1989), 493.

50. Inga Ellzey, "Concept of Medical Necessity Can Support Services When Being Audited," *Modern Medicine* (September 1, 2011), https://www.dermatology times.com.

51. Marc Berg and Geoffrey Bowker, "The Multiple Bodies of the Medical Record: Toward a Sociology of an Artifact," *Sociological Quarterly* 38, no. 3 (1997): 527.

52. "Is a Coding Audit Worth It?," The Dermatologist (website), https://www .the-dermatologist.com/article/5773.

53. Kelly-Farwell and Favreau, *Coding for Medical Necessity*, 11.

54. Kelly-Farwell and Favreau, 3.

55. Aalseth, *Medical Coding*, 98.

56. Peter R. Jensen, "A Refresher on Medical Necessity," *Family Practice Management* 13, no. 7 (2006): 28–32, available at https://www.aafp.org/fpm/2006/0700/ p28.html.

57. Jensen, "A Refresher."

58. Gregg M. Bloche, *The Hippocratic Myth: Why Doctors Are under Pressure to Ration Care, Practice Politics, and Compromise Their Promise to Heal* (New York: Palgrave MacMillan, 2011), 11.

59. Jensen, "A Refresher."

60. Foucault, *Birth of the Clinic*, 108.

61. Jensen, "A Refresher."

62. Kelly-Farwell and Favreau, *Coding for Medical Necessity*, 42.

63. Benjamin D. Smith et al., "Adoption of Intensity-Modulated Radiation Therapy for Breast Cancer in the United States," *Journal of the National Cancer Institute* 103, no. 10 (2011): 798–80.

64. Goldhill, *Catastrophic Care*, 10.

65. "Diligent Health Claim Review Service Goes Beyond Obvious Overcharges and Finds Issues with Medical Necessity," *PRWEB.COM Newswire* (February 26, 2013), http://www.digitaljournal.com.

66. See the comments on the limits of artificial intelligence and translation programs in Steven Pinker, *The Language Instinct*, 1st ed. (New York: W. Morrow & Co., 1994).

67. Derrida, *Archive Fever*, 17.

68. Derrida, 18.

69. "3M Content for Medical Necessity Validation," archived at http://www .infomedika.com/3m-coding.

70. Daniel Levinson, "Most Power Wheelchairs in the Medicare Program Did Not Meet Medical Necessity Guidelines," Department of Health and Human Services, (July 2011): 23, https://oig.hhs.gov/oei/reports/oei-04-09-00260.pdf.

71. Levinson, 15.

72. Randy Ludlow, "Dublin Pharmacists, Physician Indicted for Medicaid Fraud," *Columbus Dispatch*, July 13, 2017.

73. There are too many interesting cases to mention. With regard to rejected claims within New Mexico's Medicaid program, a state court found that the problem is not usually medically unnecessary services, but a failure to document them accurately. See Trip Jennings and Sylvia Ulloa, "The Slow-Motion Unraveling of New Mexico's Medicaid Crackdown," *New Mexico In-Depth*, June 30, 2017, http:// nmindepth.com.

74. Reed Abelson and Julie Creswell, "Hospital Chain Inquiry Cited Unnecessary Cardiac Work," *New York Times,* August 6, 2012.

75. Abelson and Creswell.

76. Janet Rehnquist, "Inpatient Hemodialysis Procedure Services Provided by Vista Del Mar Medical Group, Inc.," Department of Health and Human Services, 2001, https://oig.hhs.gov/oas/reports/region9/90100084.pdf.

77. Washington Health Alliance, "First, Do No Harm: Calculating Health

Care Waste in Washington State" (February 2018), 3, https://www.wacommunity checkup.org/media/47156/2018-first-do-no-harm.pdf.

78. Washington Health Alliance, 3.

79. Norman Daniels, *Just Health: Meeting Health Needs Fairly* (New York: Cambridge University Press, 2008), 41.

80. See, e.g., Kurt Eichenwald, "Tenet Healthcare Paying $54 Million in Fraud Settlement," *New York Times,* August 7, 2003.

81. See Deborah Stone, *Policy Paradox: The Art of Political Decision Making* (New York: W. W. Norton, 2011).

3. "No Legitimate Use"

1. See, e.g., Roy Suddaby and Royston Greenwood, "Rhetorical Strategies of Legitimacy," *Administrative Science Quarterly* 50, no. 1 (2005): 35–67.

2. David Castellon, "Medical-Marijuana Abuse: Tulare County Authorities Target Growers," *Visalia Times-Delta,* May 5, 2012.

3. As of this writing (July 2019), thirty-three states and the District of Columbia have done so, if to varying degrees. Eleven states and the District of Columbia have legalized recreational marijuana.

4. Peter A. Clark, "The Ethics of Medical Marijuana: Government Restrictions vs. Medical Necessity," *Journal of Public Health Policy* 21, no. 1 (2000): 40–60.

5. Sue Hughes, "Medical Marijuana: Where's the Evidence?," *Medscape*, July 6, 2015.

6. Janet Joy, Stanley Watson, and John Benson, "Marijuana and Medicine: Assessing the Science Base," (Washington, D.C.: Institute of Medicine, 1999), 99, https://www.ncbi.nlm.nih.gov/books/NBK230716/pdf/Bookshelf_NBK230716 .pdf. See also an analysis of the report in Kevin O'Brien and Peter A. Clark, "Case Study: Mother and Son: The Case of Medical Marijuana," *Hastings Center Report* 32, no. 5 (2002).

7. National Academy of Sciences, Committee on the Health Effects of Marijuana, "The Health Effects of Cannabis and Cannabinoids: The Current State of Evidence and Recommendations for Research," January 2017, http://www.nation alacademies.org.

8. "To Make It Harder to Get Habit Drugs," *New York Times*, January 26, 1914.

9. Controlled Substances Act, U.S.C. 21 § 812(c) (1970).

10. Comprehensive Drug Abuse Prevention and Control Act, U.S.C. 21 §§ 801–971 (2000).

11. See Annaliese Smith, "Marijuana as a Schedule I Substance: Political Ploy or Accepted Science," *Santa Clara Law Review* 40, no. 4 (1999–2000); George J. Annas, "Reefer Madness: The Federal Response to California's Medical-Marijuana Law," *New England Journal of Medicine* 337 (1997): 435–39; and George J. Annas,

"Congress, Controlled Substances, and Physician-Assisted Suicide: Elephants in Mouseholes," *New England Journal of Medicine* 354 (2006): 1079–84.

12. *United States v. Randall,* 401 U.S. 513 (1971).

13. See Mark A. Hall and Gerard F. Anderson, "Health Insurers' Assessment of Medical Necessity," *University of Pennsylvania Law Review* 140, no. 5 (1992): 1637–712.

14. Associated Press, "Four Americans Get Medical Pot from the Feds," *Associated Press News,* September 27, 2011.

15. Clinton A. Werner, "Medical Marijuana and the AIDS Crisis," *Journal of Cannabis Therapeutics* 3, no. 4 (2001): 17–33.

16. *State v. Diana,* 24 Wash. App. 908, 604 P.2d 1312 (1979).

17. *State v. Williams,* 135 Wn. 2d 365 (Wash. 1998).

18. "Last Resorts and Fundamental Rights: The Substantive Due Process Implications of Prohibitions on Medical Marijuana," *Harvard Law Review* 118, no. 6 (2005): 1985–2006.

19. *Gonzales v. Raich,* 545 US 1 (2005).

20. Miklos Pongratz, "Medical Marijuana and the Medical Necessity Defense in the Aftermath of *United States v. Oakland Cannabis Buyers' Cooperative,*" *Western New England Law Review* 25, no. 1 (2003).

21. *United States v. Oakland Cannabis Buyers' Cooperative,* 190 F.3d1109 (9th Cir. 1999).

22. Annas, "Reefer Madness," 438.

23. *United States v. Oakland Cannabis Buyers' Cooperative,* 532 U.S. 483 (2001).

24. See Aviva Halpern, "Pain: No Medical Necessity Defense for Marijuana to Controlled Substances Act," *Journal of Law, Medicine and Ethics* 29, no. 3–4 (2000): 410–11; and Alina Zanetti, "Alternative Medicine: Ninth Circuit Reverses Holding on Distribution of Medical Marijuana," *Journal of Law, Medicine and Ethics* 27, no. 4 (1998): 382–83.

25. Annas, "Reefer Madness," 439.

26. John Hudak and Grace Wallack, "Ending the U.S. Government's War on Medical Marijuana Research," Brookings Institution (website), October 20, 2015, https://www.brookings.edu.

27. J. Mitchell Pickerill and Paul Chen, "Medical Marijuana Policy and the Virtues of Federalism," *Publius: The Journal of Federalism* 38, no. 1 (2008): 22–55.

28. William Blackstone, *Commentaries on the Laws of England: A Facsimile of the First Edition of 1765–1769* (Chicago: University of Chicago Press, 1979), 120–41.

29. Michael Fleishman, "Under the Influence of Necessity," *Arizona Law Review* 45 (Spring 2003); Stephanie B. Goldberg, "Necessity Defense Fails in Massachusetts," *American Bar Association Journal* 79 (October 1993); Laurie L. Levenson, "Criminal Law: The Necessity Defense," *National Law Journal* (October 1999);

James O. Pearson Jr., "'Choice of Evils': Necessity, Duress, or Similar Defense to State or Local Criminal Charges Based on Acts of Public Protest," *American Law Reports 5th Edition* 3 (1992); Arthur Ripstein, *Equality, Responsibility, and the Law* (New York: Cambridge University Press, 1999); Laura J. Schulkind, "Applying the Necessity Defense to Civil Disobedience Cases," *New York Law Review* 64 (April 1989); Stephanie Stone, "No Surrender Requirement for Escapees Claiming Necessity Defense, Rules Texas," *West's Legal News* (January 12, 1996).

30. *Scott v. Shepherd,* 96 Eng. Rep. 525 (K.B. 1773).

31. Mary Beth Lane, "Diabetic Driver Charged in Multiple Crashes Pleads No Contest," *Columbus Dispatch,* April 16, 2011.

32. Aristotle's argument is muddled in places, but is clear in its insistence that "actions are [compulsory] when the cause is in the external circumstances and the agent contributes nothing" (Aristotle, *The Complete Works of Aristotle: The Revised Oxford Translation* [Princeton, N.J.: Princton University Press, 1984], 1110b1–3). If one is compelled externally to do something, says Aristotle, it is involuntary. This conceptual threshold requires that one attend to surrounding conditions and dispositions. He argues, for example, that a key marker of necessity is that one is never eager to do what is necessary. He exempts from responsibility those who act out of ignorance, but maintains that if one does not regret having been forced to do something unethical, then compulsion does not exclude that person from judgment, for "it is only what produces pain and regret that is *in*voluntary" (1110b16–17).

33. *United States v. Oakland Cannabis Buyers' Cooperative*, 532 U.S. 483 (2001), citing *United States v. Bailey*, 444 U.S. 394, 415 (1980).

34. Pongratz, "Medical Marijuana and the Medical Necessity Defense," 167.

35. *State v. Kurtz,* 178 Wn.2d 466, (Wash. 2013).

36. Mike Vasilinda, "Medical Marijuana," Capitol News Service, last modified April 3, 2013, http://www.flanews.com/?p=17822.

37. Shannon McFarland, "No Charges Filed against Husband in Marijuana Case," *Sarasota Herald-Tribune*, April 2, 2013, https://www.heraldtribune.com.

38. Matthew J. Seamon et al., "Medical Marijuana and the Developing Role of the Pharmacist," *American Journal of Health-System Pharmacology* 64, no. 15 (2007): 1037–44.

39. United States Department of Justice, "Attorney General Announces Formal Medical Marijuana Guidelines," news release (October 19, 2009), http://www.justice.gov/opa/pr/attorney-general-announces-formal-medical-marijuana-guidelines.

40. Josh Gerstein, "Sessions Pushes Tougher Line on Marijuana," *Politico*, February 27, 2017, http://www.politico.com.

41. New York Times Editorial Board, "Outrageous Sentences for Marijuana," *New York Times*, April 14, 2016.

42. Sally K. Richardson, Department of Health and Human Services, Letter to

State Medicaid Directors, September 4, 1998, http://downloads.cms.gov/cmsgov/archived-downloads/SMDL/downloads/SMD090498.pdf.

43. Howard Fischer, "Judge: Ahcccs Must Provide Incontinence Briefs," *Arizona Daily Sun*, May 22, 2012, https://tucson.com/news/local/article_648fa725 -39b4-5037-9d1f-bfac1473328d.html.

44. Daniel Skinner, "Defining Medical Necessity under the Patient Protection and Affordable Care Act," *Public Administration Review* 73, no. 1 (2013), S49–S59.

45. Robin K. Cohen, "Medical Necessity Definitions in Surrounding States," an OLR Research Report, January 11, 2010, https://www.cga.ct.gov/2010/rpt/2010 -R-0010.htm.

46. Rosalie Liccardo Pacula et al., "State Medical Marijuana Laws: Understanding the Laws and Their Limitations," *Journal of Public Health Policy* 23, no. 4 (2002): 413.

47. Beginning with California's Proposition 215 in 1996; see Pongratz, "Medical Marijuana and the Medical Necessity Defense," 167.

48. John Hoeffel, "Medical Marijuana Gets a Boost from Major Doctors Group," *Los Angeles Times*, November 11, 2009.

49. California Health and Safety Code, § 11362.5.

50. Kathleen T. McCarthy, "Conversations about Marijuana between Physicians and Their Patients," *The Journal of Legal Medicine* 25, no. 3 (2010): 333–49.

51. *Gonzales v. Raich*, 545 US 1 (2005).

52. Vonn Christenson, "Courts Protect Ninth Circuit Doctors Who Recommend Medical Marijuana Use," *Journal of Law, Medicine, and Ethics* 32, no. 1 (2004): 174–77.

53. Jenn Karlman, "FOX 5 Proves Medical Marijuana Card 'Easy' to Get," *FOX 5 San Diego*, April 25, 2013, http://fox5sandiego.com.

54. Norimitsu Onishi, "Marijuana Only for the Sick? A Farce, Some Angelenos Say," *The New York Times*, October, 7, 2012.

55. Josh Harkinson, "Mother Jones Writer Has a Contest with Spouse to Get Medical Marijuana Card," *Mother Jones*, October 11, 2010.

56. Gary Gibula, "Naperville Council Eyes Medical Marijuana Law," *Chicago Tribune*, November 9, 2013.

57. Madeleine Behr, "Wisconsin Legislators Seek Legalization of Medical Marijuana," *Badger Herald*, September 16, 2013.

58. J.F., "Puffs of Woe," *Economist*, October 9, 2012, http://www.economist.com.

59. Peter J. Cohen, "Medical Marijuana 2010: It's Time to Fix the Regulatory Vacuum," *Journal of Law, Medicine & Ethics* 38, no. 3 (2010): 658.

60. Cohen, 660.

61. Radley Balko, "Since Marijuana Legalization, Highway Fatalities in Colorado Are at Near-Historic Lows," *Washington Post*, August 5, 2014.

62. Angus Chen, "When Pets Do Pot: A High That's Not So Mighty," *NPR*, September 4, 2015, https://www.npr.org.

4. Contesting the Medical Necessity for Mental Health

1. Eleanore Taft, "Hundreds Expected to Walk with NAMI for Mental Health This Saturday," *Little Village*, May 5, 2017, accessed at http://littlevillagemag.com.

2. Daniel Knoepflmacher, "'Medical Necessity' in Psychiatry: Whose Definition Is It Anyway?," *Psychiatric News*, September 14, 2016.

3. Elizabeth O'Brien, "They Fought a Daughter's Heroin Addiction and Their Insurer, at the Same Time," *Time*, December 21, 2016.

4. John Turner et al., "The History of Mental Health Services in Modern England: Practitioner Memories and the Direction of Future Research," *Medical History* 59, no. 4 (2015): 599–624.

5. James E. Sabin and Norman Daniels, "Determining 'Medical Necessity' in Mental Health Practice," *Hastings Center Report* 24, no. 6 (1994): 5–13.

6. Conrad and Leiter, "Medicalization, Markets and Consumers," 170–71.

7. Louise K. Newman, "Sex, Gender and Culture: Issues in the Definition, Assessment and Treatment of Gender Identity Disorder," *Clinical Child Psychology and Psychiatry* 7, no. 3 (2002): 352–59.

8. See Daphna Stroumsa, "The State of Transgender Health Care: Policy, Law, and Medical Frameworks," *American Journal of Public Health* 104, no. 3 (2014): e31–38.

9. See Catherine Jean Archibald, "Transgender Student in Maine May Use Bathroom That Matches Gender Identity: Are Co-Ed Bathrooms Next?," *University of Missouri-Kansas City Law Review* 83 (2014): 57.

10. Thomas Szasz, *The Myth of Mental Illness: Foundations of a Theory of Personal Conduct* (New York: Harper Perennial, 1961), 40.

11. Szasz, 41. See also David A. Karp, *Speaking of Sadness: Depression, Disconnection, and the Meanings of Illness* (Oxford: Oxford University Press, 1996).

12. Conrad and Leiter, "Medicalization, Markets and Consumers," 170–71.

13. Allen Frances, "Saving Normal: An Insider's Revolt Against Out-of-Control Psychiatric Diagnosis, DSM-5, Big Pharma and the Medicalization of Ordinary Life," *Psychotherapy in Australia* 19, no. 3 (2013): 14–18.

14. Frederick C. Crews, "Talking Back to Prozac," *New York Review of Books* 54, no. 19 (2007).

15. Gerald N. Grob, "Origins of DSM-I: A Study in Appearance and Reality," *American Journal of Psychiatry* 148, no. 4 (1991): 421.

16. Paul L. Morgan et al., "Racial and Ethnic Disparities in ADHD Diagnosis from Kindergarten to Eighth Grade," *Pediatrics* 132, no. 1 (2013); Paula Caplan and

Lisa Cosgrove, eds., *Bias in Psychiatric Diagnosis* (Lanham, Md.: Jason Aronson, 2004).

17. David A. Jackson and Alan R. King, "Gender Differences in the Effects of Oppositional Behavior on Teacher Ratings of ADHD Symptoms," *Journal of Abnormal Child Psychology* 32, no. 2 (2004).

18. David H. Demmer et al., "Sex Differences in the Prevalence of Oppositional Defiant Disorder During Middle Childhood: A Meta-Analysis," *Journal of Abnormal Child Psychology* 45, no. 2 (2017): 313–25.

19. Gretchen B. LeFever, Keila V. Dawson, and Ardythe L. Morrow, "The Extent of Drug Therapy for Attention Deficit-Hyperactivity Disorder among Children in Public Schools," *American Journal of Public Health* 89, no. 9 (1999): 1362.

20. Sean Esteban McCabe, Christian J. Teter, and Carol J. Boyd, "Medical Use, Illicit Use and Diversion of Prescription Stimulant Medication," *Journal of Psychoactive Drugs* 38, no. 1 (2006): 43–56.

21. Bruce P. Dohrenwend et al., "Socioeconomic Status and Psychiatric Disorders: The Causation-Selection Issue," *Science* 255, no. 5047 (1992): 946–52.

22. Carles Muntaner et al., "Socioeconomic Position and Major Mental Disorders," *Epidemiologic Reviews* 26, no. 1 (2004): 53–62.

23. Karen Ballard and Mary Ann Elston, "Medicalisation: A Multi-Dimensional Construct," *Social Theory and Health* 3, no. 3 (2005): 228–41.

24. C. Lee Ventola, "Direct-to-Consumer Pharmaceutical Advertising: Therapeutic or Toxic?," *Pharmacy and Therapeutics* 36, no. 10 (2011): 669–74.

25. Daniel P. Carpenter, *Reputation and Power: Organizational Image and Pharmaceutical Regulation at the FDA* (Princeton, N.J.: Princeton University Press, 2010).

26. Monica J. Casper and Adele E. Clarke, "Making the Pap Smear into the 'Right Tool' for the Job: Cervical Cancer Screening in the USA, Circa 1940–95," *Social Studies of Science* 28, no. 2 (1998): 257.

27. Sabin and Daniels, "Determining 'Medical Necessity' in Mental Health Practice," 5.

28. Sabin and Daniels, 6.

29. Kenny Herzog, "Why Is It So Hard to Get Mental Health Treatment Covered by Insurance? Patients Face This Catch-22," December, 13, 2017, https://www.mic.com.

30. Sabin and Daniels, "Determining 'Medical Necessity,'" 8.

31. Sabin and Daniels, 9.

32. Sabin and Daniels, 10.

33. UnitedHealthcare, "UnitedHealthcare Medical Necessity Overview," accessed April 7, 2016, http://consultant.uhc.com/assets/medical-necessity-overview-presentation.pdf.

34. Sabin and Daniels, "Determining 'Medical Necessity,'" 5.

35. Cecilia Muñoz, "The Affordable Care Act and Expanding Mental Health Coverage," *The White House* (blog), last modified August 21, 2013, https://www .whitehouse.gov/blog/2013/08/21/affordable-care-act-and-expanding-mental -health-coverage.

36. James D. Livingston et al., "The Effectiveness of Interventions for Reducing Stigma Related to Substance Use Disorders: A Systematic Review," *Addiction* 107, no. 1 (2012): 39–50.

37. Sabin and Daniels, "Determining 'Medical Necessity' in Mental Health Practice," 5.

38. Darcy Lockman, "Is My Work 'Medically Necessary'?," *Slate.com*, January 12, 2015, https://slate.com.

39. Lockman.

40. John Mauldin, "All Smoke and No Fire? Analyzing the Potential Effects of the Mental Health Parity and Addiction Equity Act of 2008," *Law and Psychology Review* 35 (2011): 196–97.

41. *Social Security Act U.S. Code* 42 § 1396 (1935). See Daphna Stroumsa, "The State of Transgender Health Care: Policy, Law, and Medical Frameworks," *American Journal of Public Health* 104, no. 3 (2014): e31–e38.

42. Suann Kessler, "Mental Health Parity: The Patient Protection and Affordable Care Act and the Parity Definition Implications," *Hasting Science and Technology Law Journal* 6, no. 2 (2014): 145–66.

43. Patrick J. Kennedy, "With Proposed Mergers, Insurers Must Comply with Mental Health Equity Laws," *The Hill,* September 29, 2015, https://thehill.com.

44. Jenny Gold, "Is Mental Health 'Parity' Law Fulfilling Its Promise?," *CNN*, September 20, 2015, https://www.cnn.com.

45. Gold.

46. Laura Ungar and Jayne O'Donnell, "Mental Health Coverage Unequal in Many Obamacare Plans," *USA Today,* March 9, 2015.

47. Unger and O'Donnell.

48. Luhrmann, *Of Two Minds*, 10.

49. Aaron T. Beck, *Depression: Causes and Treatment* (Philadelphia: University of Pennsylvania Press, 1972). A number of other measurement tools also exist. For a brief discussion, see John W. Williams et al., "Identifying Depression in Primary Care: A Literature Synthesis of Case-Finding Instruments," *General Hospital Psychiatry* 24, no. 4 (2002): 225–37.

50. Tracy Sashidharan, Laura A. Pawlow, and Jonathan C. Pettibone, "An Examination of Racial Bias in the Beck Depression Inventory-II," *Cultural Diversity and Ethnic Minority Psychology* 18, no. 2 (2012): 203–9.

51. Judith Butler, *Bodies That Matter: On the Discursive Limits of Sex* (New York: Routledge, 2011); John B. McKinlay, "Some Contributions from the Social System to Gender Inequalities in Heart Disease," *Journal of Health and Social*

Behavior 37, no. 1 (1996): 1–26; and Anne Fausto-Sterling, *Sexing the Body: Gender Politics and the Construction of Sexuality*, 1st ed. (New York: Basic Books, 2000).

52. Thomas S. Szasz, *The Myth of Mental Illness: Foundations of a Theory of Personal Conduct* (New York: Harper Perennial, 1961), 40.

53. Ronald Pies, "Should DSM-V Designate 'Internet Addiction' a Mental Disorder?," *Psychiatry* 6, no. 2 (2009): 31–37.

54. For example, scholars have shown that the diagnosis of "drapetomania," which led to diagnostic criteria for schizophrenia, was disproportionately applied to African Americans, revealing the DSM's social and political biases, or at least blind spots, in its construction. Jack Drescher, "Out of DSM: Depathologizing Homosexuality," *Behavioral Sciences* 5, no. 4 (2015): 565–75.

55. Jonathan A. Metzl, *The Protest Psychosis: How Schizophrenia Became a Black Disease* (Boston: Beacon, 2010).

56. Center for Medicare and Medicaid Services, "Warning Signs- Plan or Policy Non-Quantitative Treatment Limitations (NQTLs) that Require Additional Analysis to Determine Mental Health Parity Compliance," https://www.cms.gov/CCIIO/Resources/Regulations-andGuidance/Downloads/MHAPEAChecklist WarningSigns.pdf.

57. Greenberg, *The Book of Woe*, 352.

58. Greenberg, 354.

59. Greenberg, 356.

60. See, e.g., Ford's response to Sabin and Daniels in William E. Ford, James E. Sabin, and Norman Daniels, "Wrong Necessity," *Hastings Center Report* 25, no. 2 (1995).

5. Reproductive Politics

1. Michel Foucault, "The Order of Discourse," 110.

2. Patton, *Rebirth of the Clinic*, xi.

3. Richard W. Wertz and Dorothy C. Wertz, *Lying-In: A History of Childbirth in America* (New York: Free Press, 1977).

4. Wertz and Wertz, 47.

5. Wertz and Wertz, 56.

6. Wertz and Wertz, 59.

7. Claudia Malacrida and Tiffany Boulton, "Women's Perceptions of Childbirth 'Choices': Competing Discourses of Motherhood, Sexuality, and Selflessness," *Gender and Society* 26, no. 5 (2012): 750.

8. See Jacqueline H. Wolf, *Deliver Me from Pain: Anesthesia and Birth in America* (Baltimore: Johns Hopkins University Press, 2009).

9. Wertz and Wertz, *Lying-In*, 25–26.

10. James E. Swain et al., "Maternal Brain Response to Own Baby-Cry Is Affected by Cesarean Section Delivery," *Journal of Child Psychology and Psychiatry* 49, no. 10 (2008): 1042–52; Catherine Deneux-Tharaux et al., "Postpartum Maternal Mortality and Cesarean Delivery," *Obstetrics & Gynecology* 108, no. 3 (2006): 541–48.

11. Marian F. MacDorman et al., "Infant and Neonatal Mortality for Primary Cesarean and Vaginal Births to Women with 'No Indicated Risk,' United States, 1998–2001 Birth Cohorts," *Birth* 33, no. 3 (2006).

12. Blue Cross Blue Shield, "Cesarean Birth Trends: Where You Live Significantly Impacts How You Give Birth," August 25, 2016, https://www.bcbs.com/sites/default/files/file-attachments/health-of-america-report/BCBS.HealthOfAmerica Report.CesareanBirthTrends.pdf.

13. See David C. Aron et al., "Variations in Risk-Adjusted Cesarean Delivery Rates According to Race and Health Insurance," *Medical Care* 38, no. 1 (2000): 35–44.

14. Lisa C. Ikemoto, "Furthering the Inquiry: Race, Class, and Culture in the Forced Medical Treatment of Pregnant Women," *Tennessee Law Review* 59, no. 3 (1992): 511.

15. Jacqueline Wolf, *Cesarean Section: An American History of Risk, Technology, and Consequence* (Baltimore: Johns Hopkins University Press, 2018), 16.

16. Patricia H. Shiono, Donald McNellis, and George G. Rhoads, "Reasons for the Rising Cesarean Delivery Rates, 1978–1984," *Obstetrics & Gynecology* 69, no. 5 (1987): 696–700.

17. Henry Chong Lee, Yasser Y. El-Sayed, and Jeffrey B. Gould, "Population Trends in Cesarean Delivery for Breech Presentation in the United States 1997–2003," *American Journal of Obstetrics and Gynecology* 199, no. 1 (2008): 59.e1–59.e8.

18. Carolyn F. Weiniger et al., "Maternal Outcomes of Term Breech Presentation Delivery: Impact of Successful External Cephalic Version in a Nationwide Sample of Delivery Admissions in the United States," *BMC Pregnancy and Childbirth* 16 (2016): 150.

19. Dhankhar Praveen, M. Mahmud Khan, and Ila M. Semenick Alam, "Threat of Malpractice Lawsuit, Physician Behavior and Health Outcomes: Testing the Presence of Defensive Medicine," *Academy of Health* (2005), available at https://www.researchgate.net/profile/M_Khan15/publication/253783054_Threat_of_Malpractice_Lawsuit_Physician_Behavior_and_Health_Outcomes_Testing_the_Presence_of_Defensive_Medicine/links/00b4953446fb06664f000000/Threat-of-Malpractice-Lawsuit-Physician-Behavior-and-Health-Outcomes-Testing-the-Presence-of-Defensive-Medicine.pdf.

20. One study found that "physicians overused cesarean delivery relative to the level that would be chosen by a financially disinterested medical provider," though the magnitude "was fairly small." Jonathan Gruber and Maria Owings, "Physician

Financial Incentives and Cesarean Section Delivery," *RAND Journal of Economics* 27, no. 1 (1996): 120.

21. William Fraser et al., "Temporal Variation in Rates of Cesarean Section or Dystocia: Does Convenience Play a Role?," *American Journal of Obstetrics and Gynecology* 156, no. 2 (1987): 300–304. See also Emmett B. Keeler and Mollyann Brodle, "Economic Incentives in the Choice between Vaginal Delivery and Cesarean Section," *Milbank Quarterly* 71, no. 3 (1993): 365–404.

22. Carey Goldberg, "NIH Rethinks Elective Caesarean Births," *Boston Globe,* March 30, 2006.

23. Michael J. Davidoff et al., "Changes in the Gestational Age Distribution among U.S. Singleton Births: Impact on Rates of Late Preterm Birth, 1992 to 2002," *Seminars in Perinatology* 30, no. 1 (2006): 8–15.

24. Theresa Morris, *Cut It Out: The C-Section Epidemic in America* (New York: New York University Press, 2013), 93. Morris, citing Declercq et al., "Listening to Mothers II: Report of the Second National U.S. Survey of Women's Childbearing Experiences" (New York: Childbirth Connection, 2006), http://www.childbirth connection.org/listeningtomothers, notes that being "overdue" was a major rhetorical warrant for declarations of medical necessity.

25. See, e.g., Keeler and Brodle, "Economic Incentives," 365–404.

26. Vahé A. Kazandjian et al., "Does a Cesarean Section Delivery Always Cost More Than a Vaginal Delivery?," *Journal of Evaluation in Clinical Practice* 3, no. 1 (2006): 16–20.

27. Gruber and Owings, "Physician Financial Incentives," 102.

28. Helen I. Marieskind, *An Evaluation of Caesarean Section in the United States: Final Report* (Washington, D.C.: United States Department of Health, Education, and Welfare, Office of the Assistant Secretary for Planning and Evaluation/ Health, 1979).

29. Morris, *Cut It Out*, 5

30. Victoria Stagg Elliott, "C-Section Rate Climbs as Options Diminish," amed news.com. Accessed September 20, 2016. This means that modes of delivery may be sensitive to geography, as in understaffed or under-resourced rural hospitals.

31. See Patt Morrison, "Too Posh to Push: Are Increased C-Sections and Induced Labors a Problem or a Right?," Southern California Public Radio KPCC, Pasadena, July 25, 2011, available at: http://www.scpr.org.

32. "NIH State-of-the-Science Conference Statement on Cesarean Delivery on Maternal Request," *NIH Consensus and State-of-the-Science Statements* 23, no. 1 (2006): 1–29.

33. Declercq et al., "Listening to Mothers II." See also Gruber and Owings, "Physician Financial Incentives," 101.

34. Jenny A. Gamble and Debra K. Creedy, "Women's Request for a Cesarean Section: A Critique of the Literature," *Birth* 27, no. 4 (2001): 263.

35. Morris, *Cut It Out*, 5.

36. Ellen S. Lazarus, "What Do Women Want?: Issues of Choice, Control, and Class in Pregnancy and Childbirth," *Medical Anthropology Quarterly* 8, no. 1 (March 1994): 25–46. Malacrida and Boulton note, "The majority of feminist research on childbirth has focused on issues of medicalization and social control," "Women's Perceptions of Childbirth 'Choices,'" 769.

37. Margaret Olivia Little et al., "Mode of Delivery: Toward Responsible Inclusion of Patient Preferences," *Obstetrics and Gynecology* 112, no. 4, (2008): 913–18.

38. Morris, *Cut It Out,* 87.

39. Morris, 89.

40. Morris, 90.

41. Shiono, McNellis, and Rhoads, "Reasons for the Rising Cesarean Delivery Rates." See also Rosalind P. Petchesky, "Fetal Images: The Power of Visual Culture in the Politics of Reproduction," *Feminist Studies* 13, no. 2 (1987): 294.

42. Morris, *Cut It Out*, 97. Morris cites "ACOG Practice Bulletin, no. 109: Intrapartum Fetal Heart Rate Monitoring: Nomenclature, Interpretation, and General Management Principles," *Obstetrics and Gynecology* 114, no. 1 (2009), 192–202.

43. Morris, *Cut It Out*, 100.

44. See Wolf, *Cesarean Section*, chapter 6, "Operating in a Culture of Risk."

45. Morris, *Cut It Out,* 106.

46. Stephanie Teleki, "Working Toward Happier Birthdays: An Effort in California to Lower C-Section Rates," *Health Affairs* (blog), November 3, 2015, https://www.healthaffairs.org.

47. Anna Gorman, "How One Hospital Reduced Unnecessary C-Sections," *The Atlantic*, May 13, 2005.

48. World Health Organization, "WHO Statement on Caesarean Section Rates: Executive Summary," April 2015, available at: http://www.who.int.

49. "NIH State-of-the-Science Conference Statement."

50. Alan L. Hillman, "Health Maintenance Organizations: Financial Incentives and Physicians' Judgments," *Annals of Internal Medicine* 112, no. 12 (1990): 891–93.

51. Morris, *Cut it Out*, 92.

52. This chapter draws on a basic argument first made in Daniel Skinner, "The Politics of Medical Necessity in American Abortion Debates," *Politics & Gender* 8, no. 1 (2012): 1–24.

53. See James C. Mohr, *Abortion in America: The Origins and Evolutions of National Policy, 1800–1900* (New York: Oxford University Press, 1978); and Daniel K. Williams, *Defenders of the Unborn* (New York: Oxford University Press, 2016).

54. Paul Adams et al., "An Open Letter to Canada's Health Minister Honourable Allan Rock," *Canadian Physicians for Life*, http://www.physiciansforlife.ca/html/conscience/articles/openletter.html.

55. Laura Purdy, "Medicalization, Medical Necessity, and Feminist Medicine," *Bioethics* 15, no. 3 (2001): 256.

56. Gruber and Owings, "Physician Financial Incentives," 101.

57. Petchesky, Rosalind P., *Abortion and Woman's Choice: The State, Sexuality, and Reproductive Freedom*, rev. ed. (Boston: Northeastern University Press, 1990), 289.

58. *Roe v. Wade*, 410 U.S. 113 (1973).

59. Petchesky, *Abortion and Woman's Choice*, 289.

60. Petchesky, 268.

61. *Doe v. Bolton*, 410 U.S. 179, 192 (1973).

62. In some cases, this created a black market of necessity certificates for patients who cannot get them from doctors. See Dale Lezon, "Sugar Land Man Pleads Guilty in Medicare Fraud Case," *Houston Chronicle*, August 24, 2010, http://www.chron.com.

63. *Maher v. Roe*, 432 U.S. 464 (1977).

64. Willard Cates Jr., "The Hyde Amendment in Action: How Did the Restriction of Federal Funds for Abortion Affect Low-Income Women?," *JAMA* 246, no. 10 (1981): 1109–12.

65. Linda Greenhouse and Reva B. Siegel, eds. *Before Roe v. Wade: Voices that Shaped the Abortion Debate before the Supreme Court's Ruling* (New York: Kaplan Publishing, 2010), 264.

66. *Roe v. Wade*, 410 U.S. 113 (1973).

67. *Stenberg v. Carhart,* 530 U.S. 916 (2000).

68. *Gonzales v. Carhart*, 550 U.S. 124 (2007).

69. George J. Annas, "The Supreme Court and Abortion Rights," *New England Journal of Medicine* 356, no. 21 (2007): 2201–7.

70. *Gonzales v. Carhart.*

71. John Stuart Mill, *A System of Logic, Ratiocinative and Inductive: Being a Connected View of the Principles of Evidence and the Methods of Scientific Investigation* (New York: Harper, 1884); Daniel C. Dennett, *The Intentional Stance* (Cambridge, Mass: MIT Press, 1987).

72. Lantos, *The Lazarus Case*, 7.

73. Amendment to H.R. 3962, as reported. Offered by Mr. Stupak of Michigan and Mr. Pitts of Pennsylvania, http://housedocs.house.gov/rules/3962/Stupak 3962_108.pdf.

74. George J. Annas, "Abortion Politics and Health Insurance Reform," *New England Journal of Medicine* 361, no. 27 (2009): 2589–91.

75. Petchesky, *Abortion and Woman's Choice*, 289.

76. *Planned Parenthood of Southeastern Pennsylvania v. Casey*, 505 U.S. 833 (1992). February 2011 saw a new front open when Republicans announced their intention to redefine rape, which would have the effect of limiting those cases that

could be included in the exceptions offered under abortion bans. See Sady Doyle, "John Boehner's Push to Redefine Rape," *Salon.com*, February 1, 2011, https://www.salon.com; Ann Coulter, "Prescriptions for Disaster Now Covered under Obamacare," *TownHall.com*, March 31, 2010, https://townhall.com.

77. Two exemplars are Kenneth Burke, *A Rhetoric of Motives* (Berkeley: University of California Press, 1950), and Stanley Fish, *Doing What Comes Naturally* (Durham, N.C.: Duke University Press, 1990).

78. See Rachel K. Jones and Jenna Jerman, "Abortion Incidence and Service Availability in the United States, 2014," *Perspectives on Sexual and Reproductive Health* 49, no. 1, (2017): 17–27.

79. Reuters, "Woman Gets 20-Year Sentence in Attacks on Abortion Clinics," *The New York Times*, September 9, 1995.

80. Ron Sylvester, "Scott Roeder Gets Hard 50 in Murder of Abortion Provider George Tiller," *Wichita Eagle*, updated October 24, 2014, https://www.kansas.com.

81. Morris, *Cut It Out*, 17.

Conclusion

1. Foucault, *Power/Knowledge*, 87.

2. Andrew Ward, "Needs, Medical Necessity, and the Problem of Helping the Uninsured," *Theoria: A Journal of Social & Political Theory* 54, no. 112 (2007): 85.

3. Morreim, "The Futility of Medical Necessity," 25.

4. Morriem, 25.

5. Kenneth J. Arrow, "Uncertainty and the Welfare Economics of Medical Care," *American Economic Review* 53, no. 5 (1963): 941–73. For an update on the debate about symmetry in knowledge on health care markets, see Deborah Haas-Wilson, "Arrow and the Information Market Failure in Health Care: The Changing Content and Sources of Health Care Information," *Journal of Health Politics, Policy and Law* 26, no. 5 (2001): 1031–44.

6. *Varnum v. Thruston*, 17 Md. 470, 496, 1861 WL 2156 (1861) characterizes *contra proferentem* as a doctrine of "strictness and rigor, and not to be resorted to but where other rules of exposition fail."

7. *Economy Premier Assurance Company Co. v. Western National Mutual Insurance Company*, 839 N.W.2d 749 (Minn. Ct. App. 2013). See also Steven Plitt, "Historical Tour of the Contra Proferentem Doctrine," *Claims Journal*, April 28, 2014, at http://www.claimsjournal.com. However, as *Catlin Specialty Insurance Company v. QA3 Financial Corp.*, 2014 WL 2990520 (S.D.N.Y. July 2, 2014), held, *contra proferentem* loses some of its force when the insured is a relatively sophisticated party, such as a company with a legal staff, or in light of other "extrinsic evidence."

8. Omri Ben-Shahar, "Fixing Unfair Contracts," *Stanford Law Review* 63, no. 869 (2011): 877.

9. Morreim recounts specific instances in E. Haavi Morreim, *Holding Health Care Accountable: Law and the New Medical Marketplace* (New York: Oxford University Press, 2001).

10. *Loyola University of Chicago v. Humana Insurance Company* marked a turning point as the Seventh Circuit of the U.S. Court of Appeals held, "Although it seems callous for Humana to deny coverage for a life-saving procedure [a heart transplant that lacked Humana's prior approval] and thereafter deny all subsequent hospital expenses—in essence saying to [the patient], 'we will not cover you because you should be dead'—Humana's humanity is not the issue here. This is a contract case and the language of the benefit plan controls." *Loyola University of Chicago v. Humana Insurance Company*, 996 F.2d 895, 903 (7th Cir. 1993). Quoted in Morreim, "The Futility of Medical Necessity," 23–24.

11. Maxwell Gregg Bloche, "Trust and Betrayal in the Medical Marketplace," *Stanford Law Review* 55, no. 3 (2002): 953.

12. Carole Pateman and Charles W. Mills, *Contract and Domination*, 1st ed. (Cambridge U.K.: Polity, 2007).

13. See, e.g., George Loewenstein et al., "Consumers' Misunderstanding of Health Insurance," *Journal of Health Economics* 32, no. 5 (2013): 850–62; and George Loewenstein and Saurabh Bhargava, "The Simple Case against Health Insurance Complexity," *NEJM Catalyst*, August 23, 2016.

14. Sonia Corrêa, Rosalind P. Petchesky, and Richard Parker, *Sexuality, Health and Human Rights* (New York: Routledge, 2008), 152.

15. Corrêa, Petchesky, and Parker, 153.

16. Corrêa, Petchesky, and Parker, 153.

17. Stone, *Policy Paradox*, 349.

18. Stone, 353.

19. Corrêa, Petchesky, and Parker, *Sexuality, Health and Human Rights,* 155.

20. Butler, *Bodies That Matter, Sexuality, Health and Human Rights,* 152.

21. Bloche, *Hippocratic Myth*, 81.

22. Casper and Clarke, "Making the Pap Smear into the 'Right Tool' for the Job," 257.

23. See Corrêa, Petchesky, and Parker, *Sexuality, Health and Human Rights,* 161.

24. Jacques Derrida, "Force of Law: 'The Mystical Foundation of Authority,'" in *Deconstruction and the Possibility of Justice*, ed. Drucilla Cornell, Michel Rosenfeld, and David Carlson (New York: Routledge, 1992).

25. See "The Question Concerning Technology," in Martin W. Lewis, *Green Delusions: An Environmentalist Critique of Radical Environmentalism* (Durham, N.C.: Duke University Press, 1992).

26. Susan R. Drossman, Elisa R. Port, and Emily B. Sonnenblick, "Why the Annual Mammogram Matters," *New York Times*, October 28, 2015.

27. Elisabeth Rosenthal, "Breast Cancer Chemo Is Often Unnecessary—But Doctors May Not Want You to Know," *Fortune*, September 7, 2018.

28. See David H. Newman, "Ignoring the Science on Mammograms," *New York Times,* November 28, 2012.

29. See U.S. Preventive Services Task Force, *Final Recommendation Statement: Breast Cancer: Screening,* January 2016, https://www.uspreventiveservicestaskforce .org.

30. Susanne B. Haga and Huntington F. Willard, "Defining the Spectrum of Genome Policy," *Nature Reviews Genetics* 7, no. 12 (2006): 969.

31. Eric Klein, "Medicare Considers Coverage of Genetic Prostate Cancer Test," *Cleveland Clinic Health Essentials,* June 8, 2015, https://health.clevelandclinic.org.

32. National Institutes of Health, "Estimates of Funding for Various Research, Condition, and Disease Categories," last modified May 18, 2018, https://report.nih .gov/categorical_spending.aspx.

33. The U.K. is also heavily invested in this line of research, suggesting an international trend. See Fergus Walsh, "DNA Mapping for Cancer Patients," BBC News (website), December 10, 2012, https://www.bbc.com.

34. "The Precision Medicine Initiative," *The White House* (blog), https://obama whitehouse.archives.gov.

35. Mike Miliard, "NIH Precision Medicine Project to Explore Enrollment of Kids," *HealthcareITNews,* July 20, 2017, http://www.healthcareitnews.com/news/ nih-precision-medicine-project-explore-enrollment-kids.

36. Rishona L. Mackoff et al., "Attitudes of Genetic Counselors Towards Genetic Susceptibility Testing in Children," *Journal of Genetic Counseling* 19, no. 4 (2010): 402–16.

37. Chad Terhune, "Health Net Faces Suit over Refusals to Cover Treatments," *Los Angeles Times,* September 13, 2012.

38. Kerry Hannon, "New Rules on Wellness Programs Spark Privacy Worries," *Forbes,* May 29, 2016.

39. Vanderpool, Donna. "HIPAA: Should I Be Worried?," *Innovations in Clinical Neuroscience* 9, no. 11–12 (2012): 51–55.

40. "The Question Concerning Technology," in Martin Heidegger, *Basic Writings: From Being and Time (1927) to The Task of Thinking (1964),* ed. David Farrell Krell (San Francisco: Harper, 1993), 307–41.

41. Dion Farquhar, *The Other Machine: Discourse and Reproductive Technologies,* 1st ed. (New York: Routledge, 1996), 65.

42. Nietzsche noticed this dynamic in his observation that "science today is a *hiding place* for every kind of discontent." Friedrich Nietzsche, *On the Genealogy of Morals and Ecco Homo,* trans. Walter Kaufmann (New York: Vintage Books, 1989), 147.

43. UnitedHealthcare, "UnitedHealthcare Medical Necessity Overview," https://www.uhctools.com/assets/M50195-B%20Member%20FAQs%20Medical%20Necessity.pdf.

44. For a complete list, see Aetna, "Complementary and Alternative Medicine," last review June 19, 2019, http://www.aetna.com/cpb/medical/data/300_399/0388.html.

45. Sara Rosenbaum et al., *Medical Necessity in Private Health Plans: Implications for Behavioral Health Care* (Rockville, Md.: United States Department of Health and Human Services, Substance Abuse and Mental Health Services Administration, 2003), 13.

46. Trisha Greenhalgh, Jeremy Howick, and Neal Maskrey, "Evidence Based Medicine: A Movement in Crisis?," *BMJ* 348 (2014): g3725.

47. Aristotle, *Aristotle's Treatise on Rhetoric*, trans. Thomas Hobbes, 2nd ed. (Oxford: D. A. Talboys, 1833).

48. See, e.g., Krzysztof J. Gorgolewski and Russell A. Poldrack, "A Practical Guide for Improving Transparency and Reproducibility in Neuroimaging Research," *PLOS Biology* 14, no. 7 (2016): e1002506.

49. Philip Selznick, *Leadership in Administration: A Sociological Interpretation* (Evanston, Ill.: Row, Peterson, 1957), 17.

50. Ruger, *Health and Social Justice*, 207.

51. Sabin and Daniels, "Determining 'Medical Necessity' in Mental Health Practice," 12.

52. Sabin and Daniels, 12.

53. Derrida, "Force of Law: 'The Mystical Foundation of Authority.'"

54. In law, see Gerald B. Wetlaufer, "Rhetoric and Its Denial in Legal Discourse," *Virginia Law Review* 76, no. 8 (1990): 1545–97; in economics, Deirdre N. McCloskey, *The Rhetoric of Economics*, 2nd ed. (Madison: University of Wisconsin Press, 1998).

55. Bloche, *Hippocratic Myth*, 58.

56. Bloche, 59.

57. Tara Bannow, "Hospitals Cry Foul and Sue Anthem Over New Policies," *Modern Healthcare*, April 21, 2018.

58. Sabin and Daniels, "Determining 'Medical Necessity' in Mental Health Practice," 13.

59. American Medical Association, "Medical Necessity and Due Process," American Medical Association Model Managed Care Contract: Supplement 1, http://www.montgomerymedicine.org/members/learningdocs/AMA%20Medical%20Necessity.pdf.

60. See *Vox.com* health care reporter Sarah Kliff's year-long project to collect emergency room bills, at https://www.vox.com/2018/2/27/16936638/er-bills-emergency-room-hospital-fees-health-care-costs.

61. See, for example, David Gollaher, *Circumcision: A History of the World's Most Controversial Surgery* (New York: Basic Books, 2000), 114.

62. Daniel Skinner, "Defining Medical Necessity under the Patient Protection and Affordable Care Act," *Public Administration Review* 73, no. S1 (2013): S49–S59.

63. For a discussion of IPAB, see Timothy Stoltzfus Jost, "The Independent Payment Advisory Board," *New England Journal of Medicine* 363 (2010): 103–5.

64. "GAO Study and Report on Determination and Implementation of Payment and Coverage Policies under the Medicare Program," U.S. Code 42 (2012), § 1395kkk, https://www.govinfo.gov.

65. Ben Kamisar, Melanie Zanona, and Cristina Marcos, "Trump Signs Budget Deal Ending Shutdown," *The Hill*, February 9, 2018, https://thehill.com.

66. In Canada, the idea of establishing a two-tier system (as exists in the U.K.) is raised from time to time as a way of alleviating public resources, but has thus far been dismissed. See John E. Wennberg, "Medical Necessity and the Debate over [Expletive Deleted] Care," *Public Health Reports* 112, no. 4 (1997): 306–7; and an exchange in Carolyn A. DeCoster and Marni D. Brownell, "DeCoster and Brownell Reply," *Public Health Reports* 112, no. 6 (1997): 301.

67. See Ann Silversides, "Canada Health Act Breaches Are Being Ignored, Pro-Medicare Groups Charge," *Canadian Medical Association Journal* 179, no. 11 (2008): 1112–13.

68. Cathy Charles and colleagues argue that contests over the meaning of medical necessity in Canada proliferated in the 1990s to refine the scope of care and protect Canada's fledgling health care system. Charles et al., "Medical Necessity in Canadian Health Policy."

69. Unfortunately, there are signs that distrust in government is on the rise in Canada. "Majority of Canadians Distrust Government: Poll Suggests," CBC Radio (website), February 16, 2017, http://www.cbc.ca.

70. David Baker and Faisal Bhabha, "Universality and Medical Necessity: Statutory and Charter Remedies to Individual Claims to Ontario Health Insurance Funding," *Health Law Review* 13, no. 1 (2004): 25.

71. Baker and Bhabha, 25.

72. Neoliberal developments are also undermining the social cohesion that made Canadian health care unique. This process, however, as with Canadian politics itself, is uneven, with stark differences in system maintenance between provinces. See Ken McGeorge, "Public Confidence in Health System Is Being 'Eroded,'" CBC News (website), August 27, 2014, https://www.cbc.ca.

73. Wennberg, "Medical Necessity and the Debate over [Expletive Deleted] Care," 302.

74. Daniel Skinner, Berkeley Franz, and Kelly Kelleher, "What Challenges Do Appalachian Non-Profit Hospitals Face in Taking on Community Health

Needs Assessments? A Qualitative Study from Ohio," *Journal of Rural Health* 34, no. 2 (2018): 182–92.

75. Charles et al., "Medical Necessity in Canadian Health Policy," 388.

76. Susan Edgman-Levitan and Tejal Gandhi, "Empowering Patients as Partners in Health Care," *Health Affairs Blog*, July 24, 2014, https://www.healthaffairs.org.

77. See the NIH funding call for the study "Marijuana, Prescription Opioid, or Prescription Benzodiazepine Drug Use among Older Adults," Department of Health and Human Services, National Institutes of Health, https://grants.nih.gov/grants/guide/pa-files/PA-17-198.html.

78. Kevin P. Hill and Andrew J. Saxon, "The Role of Cannabis Legalization in the Opioid Crisis," *JAMA Internal Medicine* 178, no. 5 (2018): 679–80.

79. Alex Spiegel, "How a Bone Disease Grew to Fit the Prescription," *NPR*, December 21, 2009, http://www.npr.org.

80. For a criticism of the concept of prediabetes, see Isabel Beshar and Hank Campbell, "Prediabetes: The Epidemic That Never Was, and Shouldn't Be," *Chicago Tribune*, July 29, 2016.

81. Arthur Kleinman, Leon Eisenberg, and Byron Good, "Culture, Illness and Care: Clinical Lessons from Anthropologic and Cross-Cultural Research," *Annals of Internal Medicine* 88, no. 2 (1978): 251–58.

82. Gerard Anderson and James R. Knickman, "Changing the Chronic Care System to Meet People's Needs," *Health Affairs* 20, no. 6 (2001): 146–60.

83. David Mechanic, "The Managed Care Backlash: Perceptions and Rhetoric in Health Care Policy and the Potential for Health Care Reform," *Milbank Quarterly* 79, no. 1 (2001): 46.

84. Dhruv Khullar, "Do You Trust the Medical Profession?" *New York Times,* January 23, 2018.

85. See, e.g., Bloche, "Trust and Betrayal in the Medical Marketplace," 919–49.

86. As Burke explains, "In being identified with B, A is 'substantially one' with a person other than himself. Yet at the same time he remains unique, an individual locus of motives. Thus, he is both joined and separate, at once a distinct substance and consubstantial with another." Kenneth Burke, *A Rhetoric of Motives* (Berkeley: University of California Press, 1969), 21.

87. Susan Miller, *Trust in Texts: A Different History of Rhetoric* (Carbondale: Southern Illinois University Press, 2008).

88. Foucault, "The Order of Discourse," 119.

89. Wittgenstein, *Philosophical Investigations*, sec. 241.

90. Bloche, *Hippocratic Myth*.

91. Richard Hofstadter, *The Paranoid Style in American Politics, and Other Essays* (New York: Vintage Books, 2008).

Index

Healthcare Common Procedure Coding System, 54
health care reform, 6, 27, 143, 173, 176
Health Insurance Portability and Accountability Act, 54, 163
health maintenance organization, 40, 155. *See also* insurance companies
HHS. *See* United States Department of Health and Human Services
HIPAA. *See* Health Insurance Portability and Accountability Act
HMO. *See* health maintenance organization
Holder, Eric, 91
Hospital Corporation of America, 74
human rights. *See under* rights
Hyde Amendment, 139–40, 143. *See also* abortion

ICD. *See* International Classification of Diseases, Injuries, and Causes of Death
IMRT. *See* intensity-modulated radiation therapy
Independent Payment Advisory Board, 173, 213
informed consent, 35, 36–37, 170, 171
Institute of Medicine. *See* National Academy of Medicine
insurance, 6, 7, 14, 18, 26–28, 37–40, 54–56, 76, 113, 122, 160, 162; and the Mental Health Parity and Addiction Equity Act, 106–7
insurance companies, 30, 40, 105, 117–19, 155. *See also* appeals
intensity-modulated radiation therapy, 70
International Classification of Diseases, Injuries, and Causes of Death, 48, 53–54, 56, 59, 61, 67, 69

internet: and coding, 49, 56, 70; and patient knowledge, 63, 171
IPAB. *See* Independent Payment Advisory Board

Jensen, Peter, 68–69

Kelly-Farwell, Deborah, 55, 60
Knoepflmacher, Daniel, 27, 105
Kurtz, William, 89–90

language games. *See under* Wittgenstein, Ludwig
Lantos, John, 31, 35, 64–65
Leiter, Valerie, 109
libertarianism, 24, 38, 152–53, 179
Lockman, Darcy, 117–18
Lou Gehrig's disease. *See* amyotrophic lateral sclerosis
Luhrmann, T. M., 51, 55–56, 119

Maher v. Roe, 139
malpractice, 14, 28, 35, 64–65, 71, 132, 133, 145–46
managed care organizations (MCO), 30. *See also* insurance companies
marijuana, 17–18, 79–103; and ballot initiatives, 84, 95, 100, 101; and chronic pain, 2–3, 81, 85, 89, 92, 101; compassionate use of, 85, 95, 98; federal laws, 82, 84, 86, 96; medical and recreational legalization of, 80–81, 90, 99–101; state laws, 87, 91–96. *See also* Controlled Substances Act; National Organization for the Reform of Marijuana Laws
Mechanic, David, 179
Medicaid, 3, 5, 32, 60, 93, 94, 115, 118, 172
medicalization, 71, 158, 163–64, 177; abortion and, 139–40; childbirth

DANIEL SKINNER is associate professor of health policy in the Department of Social Medicine at Ohio University's Heritage College of Osteopathic Medicine in Dublin, Ohio. He is the coeditor of *Not Far from Me: Stories of Opioids and Ohio*. He is codirector of the Osteopathic Health Policy fellowship, director of the Comparative Health Systems–Cuba program at Ohio University, and host of Prognosis Ohio, a biweekly podcast about health policy and politics in Ohio.